THE TUSCANY EXPRESS (REVISED)

By

DEIRDRE MCNAMARA, D. HOM

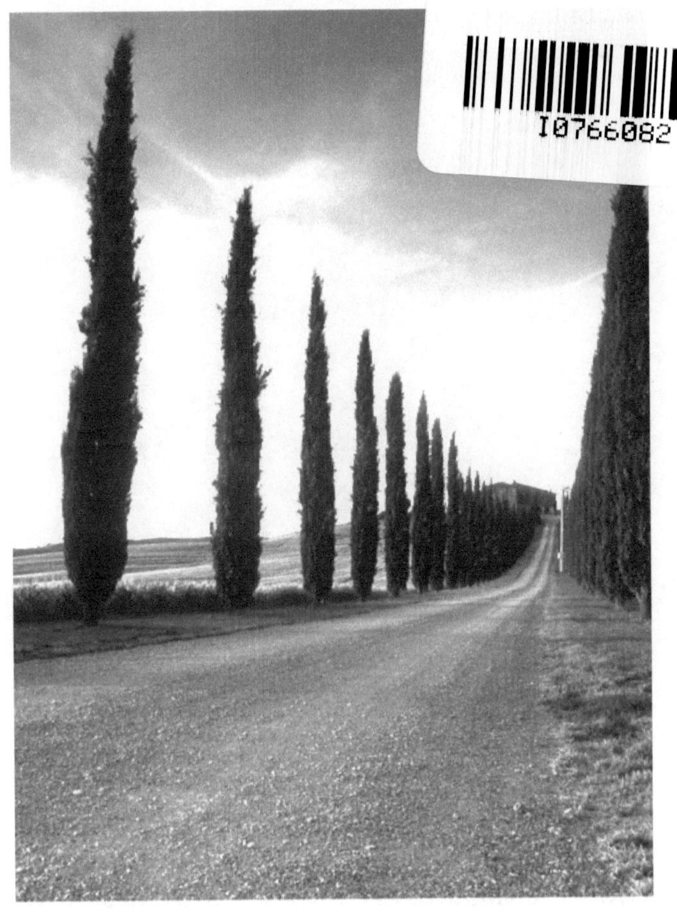

One of the most humble, and yet most powerful instruments of God's "arsenal of healing…" the ubiquitous Dandelion. DM

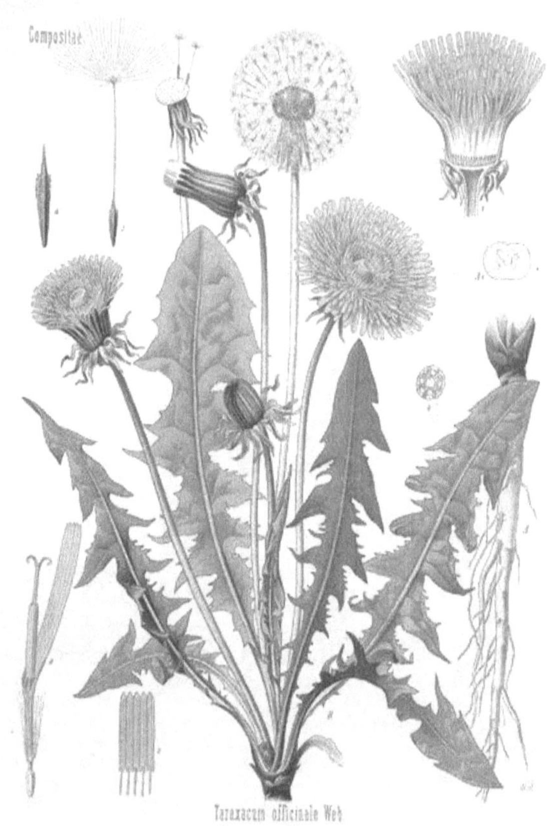

THE TUSCANY EXPRESS" IS DEDICATED TO THE GREAT HAHNEMANNIANS PAST AND PRESENT - GRATITUDE TO DR. MARGARET TYLER, DR. MARJORIE BLACKIE, GREAT ENGLISH WOMEN HOMOEOPATHISTS - AND TO MY DEDICATED FRIENDS IN ORTHODOXY, WHO SHARE THE SAME DESIRE TO RELIEVE HUMAN SUFFERING. ABOVE ALL, TO YOUNG NICCOLO.

SIMILIA SIMILIBUS CURENTER![1]

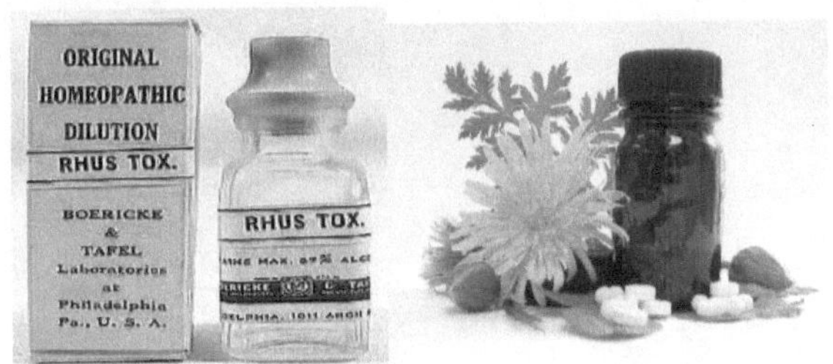

Let likes cure like! Fundamental principal of Homeopathy.

© 2019 DEIRDRE MCNAMARA, NICCOLO MCNAMARA

THE TUSCANY EXPRESS (REVISED) 2ND EDITION

In memoriam Lionel Roy Ogden, MBE, Homeopath.

Foreword

"The Tuscany Express" (Revised) is an account of some situations encountered by the Homeopath, off duty, far from home, and practice, on vacation, or assignement. It shows the effectiveness of Homeopathy, expertly practiced in less than ideal situations. Hopefully it will provide some insight into the precision of Homeopathy and the suffering it relieves without further taxing an already stressed bio-immune system

"The Tuscany Express" contains no case histories of registered patients. As some of the contingencies dealt with have been in emergency situations, detailed notes are not available, so 'The Tuscany Express' should not be considered a text book or primer on, say, chronic cases.

It does, however, demonstrate that homeopathy can be used in crisis situations and in keeping with the light hearted nature of the book, a list of remedies used is provided at the conclusion of the book, but scrambled so that the serious student may draw his/her conclusions independently, if interested.

INDEX

THE TUSCANY EXPRESS (Italy)

I was on the Express from Firenze (Florence) to Bologna, travelling through the amazing Tuscan landscape, returning to my wonderful Star Vespucci Hotel outside Florence, when a young man walked rapidly down the corridor, looking into all the compartments and calling for a 'doctor.'

I introduced myself as a Homeopathist and offered my help should an orthodox physician not be available. As a guest in Italy I did not want to cause any offense to local medics nor injury to the good name of Homeopathy.

The young man said, 'per piacere,' and guided me to a carriage a few 'doors' back, where a man in his late forties was huddled in fetal position on the seat, groaning with pain.

There were a number of people outside, and a couple of relatives inside. The young man introduced himself as a paramedic. I'll call him 'Angelo.'

He suspected the gentleman was experiencing a cardiac episode or arrest.

I asked for all but one relative to wait outside, and for a window to be opened and to loosen his clothing. His face was 'puffy,' feet and abdomen swollen, eyes yellow, somewhat bloodshot and bleary. I then took his pulses – as in 'Oriental' pulses, found anomalies on the Cardiac pulse; it was weak, intermittent and 'thready.' However his liver pulse was pounding. Yes, his friends confirmed that they were partying all night. For that, I'll call him Sg. Fiesta.

For that and other indications, I provided one dose of the *indicated remedy*, waited to see if the 'picture' would clear or improve, and within *minutes* was glad to see he was sitting up and ready to continue his journey.

His friends all crowded to the door, and cheered - most knew about Homeopathy, and were vocal in their support! I had many invitations for libations from the generous Italians, but declined for reasons of protocol. I might accept those invitations today, however!!!

The Paramedic, Angelo, had judiciously called ahead to the nearest hospital, and after some wrangling, Sg Fiesta (Mr. 'Party man') very reluctantly agreed to break his journey and go to hospital for tests.

The train made an unscheduled stop. The ambulance was waiting at the station while a team of paramedics were waiting *on the platform with a gurney, or wheeled stretcher, all exquisitely and calmly organized.*

An hour or so later, the Paramedic returned to my carriage to advise me that the hospital had contacted him to confirm that blood tests were positive for cardiac arrest but that he was well enough to travel back to Bologna later that evening.

I know of no other health care system that is as compassionate and efficient as that encountered in Italy on the Tuscany Express.

Italy would be well to maintain their standards and not allow their Emergency Rooms* to become ghastly images of the cruel New York model, where so many foreign physicians go to train.

Ireland has managed – despite or because of intense mismanagement** – to short change her hospitals. Now even the one sure "cure" has gone away with wisdom – the diagnostic cup of tea.

If you're well enough to drink it, you can't be that sick,

If you refuse it – "we'll get the doctor in to see you right away…"

Still, when the Irish ran their own hospitals, the ER rooms (A and E) may have had limited equipment, but they were always clean and mostly kind, a far cry from the hysteria, noise and clutter of New York's ERs.

I hope Italy has maintained her standards since the publication of the First Edition of the Tuscany Express.

- Update: In 2018 I accompanied a sick young man to an ER near Malpensa Airport. He was unwell after a transatlantic flight. For hours, they ignored my request for re-hydration and Oxygen, and frankly reminded me of the dread New York model. My worst fears were realized.
- Finally when they acceded to my request for hydration, the young man quickly recovered. Flying can be very stressful for certain constitutions.
- In Ireland, in order to impress the EU moguls, the Irish government, under Bertie Ahern took money from the Hospitals in order to build and update sports arenas.

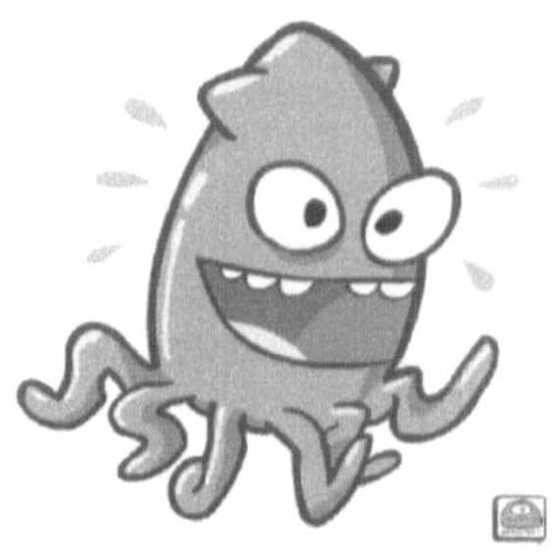

THE MUSICIAN AND THE PLATE OF CALAMARI (NYC)

If only they had told me about the Calamari at the outset.

It would not have changed the remedy.

It would have saved a visit to the Emergency Room.

A friend called to say his son was in distress. I don't usually respond to calls from persons not registered as patients, but I'd seen him grow up, and knew the family quite well.

It was a similar scenario to Sg Fiesta. Patient lying on the couch, groaning with pain, posterior left from lower angle of scapula to just above his waist line on the right.

I saw his grandmother with acute cholecystitis (gall bladder attack) just as the medics arrived to take her for emergency surgery. Suspected either a family weakness or family tendency to rich and fatty foods, but we never presume.

I am certain that Homeopathy would have "cancelled" her need for surgery, but myprofessional services were not required – just my 'comforting' presence…but that's another story. The poor woman was relentlessly cold, shaking under heavy blankets. (Sepia, Arsenicum A, Nux v, etc)

Back to *hard working,* much *travelled* Mr. RockBand!

I immediately thought of Nux Vomica, but did a quick anamnesis to see if another remedy 'peeked' through' the symptoms.   The Pulse Diagnoses and concomitant symptoms confirmed a 'full ropey pulse' on the Gall Bladder meridian.

Indicated remedy - one dose only.

I was certain that Mr. RB avoided the alcohol and drugs associated with the entertainment industry and was otherwise healthy, so was puzzled by the severity of the attack.

Patient responded very quickly, so I returned to my apartment.

At 7 am the following morning I received another call.

Mr. RB had another attack, had spent the night in the ER of New York Hospital but they could not determine whether the pain originated in his kidney or gall bladder so they sent him home.

I dressed quickly and returned to their apartment. Mr. RB's pain had subsided somewhat but was still intrusive. Suddenly I spotted a dish on the coffee table – a *giant dish of deep fried calamari!!!*

Please skip the fried foods if your family has a history of gall bladder or liver disease if you don't want surgery. Authentic Homeopaths are thin on the ground…

And yes, he'd scarfed down a plate-load before my first visit and was *feeling so much better after the Indicated Remedy that he started on a second portion…hence the second episode. This quickly and finally resolved to a second dose of the same remedy.*

Now this always puzzles me.

When a Homeopathist performs spectacularly or well, it's taken for granted but outside our beloved registered patients we are seldom given second chances.

For instance, the young man sat in the ER for hours *in agony,* while an army of highly paid staff took bloods, made X rays, poked, prodded, etc., and ultimately did nothing. Cost to insurance companies = thousands of dollars. Result = Zilch, Nothing, Nada!

Homeopathy initially cured the man within minutes, but I was not called back when his symptoms returned. Nor was an honest answer given when I asked if he had 'eaten anything unusual' that night.

If we start charging thousands of dollars for a visit – which Homeopathy is actually worth - we might engender more respect. On the other hand, we would miss so many wonderful patients and friends.

And I did 'break the rules,' re treating persons who were not committed to Homeopathy - so I can't really complain. The wisdom of the historic Homeopathists triumphs in this regard!

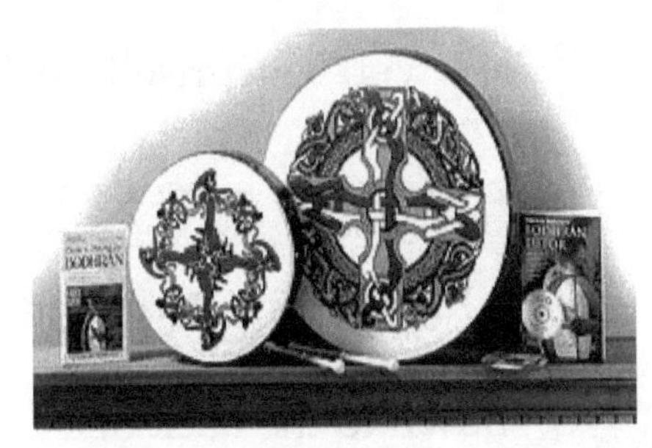

"SUFFERING IRISH…" (CT, USA)

My late husband, actor producer Dermot McNamara, was invited to visit Tom and Pat King's house in Connecticut. It wasn't their own property but a house that Tom was living in while reconstructing it. Unknown to us, but in retrospect not too surprising, was the fact that it was a stealth base for extreme Irish nationalists. We were lured there for the purposes of providing, for neither money nor respect, our expertise to a bunch of yobos who had stolen Dermot's theatre with the help and support of NY's far left City Council President Paul O'Dwyer, and who were also very well funded.

We were surprised to be picked up by a man under sentence of execution by the Official IRA for stealing millions from Bernadette Devlin's campaign funds, and shown to the back of a converted Post Office van. After a long, harrowing journey during which my imagination ran wild, we eventually pulled up outside a very nice Connecticut House complete with stables and paddock, unfolded our stiff limbs and breathed what was now the fresh, night air.

Pat, an ex nun, and Tom, a red headed 'viking,' gave us a snack and showed us to a nice room where we fell into a welcome, deep and profound sleep...

...shattered at an unearthly hour by the sound of a bodhran* outside our window and the chant: 'Suffering Irish, suffering Irish, suffering Irish Cath-o-lic!'

The tone of that chant made it very clear that the IRA were not invested in 'defending' or 'protecting' Catholicism in Northern Ireland.

They told us they were raising money for the 'Green Cross,' and were doing a street pageant based on Celtic legend at Lincoln Center.

A friend of Dermot's, a former owner of the Irish Pavilion, and sympathetic to the Provisional IRA later hissed 'I don't care what they tell you about band-aids and blankets – it's going for fookin' guns!'

And yet they received public grants denied to the Irish Players.

The 'pageant' gave them the 'background' to steal Dermot's theatre right from under his nose.

Suffering Irish indeed!

The rest of that story belongs elsewhere, but the memory of that chant echoed in my mind when I entered the refectory or dining room of a community of recovering drug addicts from around the world. Posted on the wall was a sign with the words: 'SUFFER. SWALLOW. SILENCE' or 'SWALLOW, SUFFER, SILENCE.'

They might as well have put 'Lasciate Ogni Speranza voi ch'entrate!'* Any sequence was ominous!

The addicts, many of them ill and infected with Hepatitis A, B, C slept in bunk beds, four to a small room. Bathrooms were limited and they were obligated to eat everything placed on their plate regardless of size or quality.

Since much of the food was experimental – eg, they were learning to make cheese from the milk of their donated cow – which some-how fermented, but was still forced upon them, the consequences were sometimes dire and the bathrooms in full use.

Given that they lived 'on providence,' ie, donations, and were not permitted to ask for staples such as bathroom tissue, paper towels, etc., they were assured of considerable further suffering.

Only 15% were Irish, despite the fact that the majority of donations came from Irish philanthropists.

***

They were caught between two stools: they were a community that lived a monastic, highly structured and penitential lifestyle, but they were *not* a religious community.

They were a group of recovering drug addicts under strict controls from their founder, Mother Elvira, but *under no local or national regulation.*

They were obliged to live 'on Providence' – while handsome donations went to the motherhouse.

Persons wanting to be formally involved, e.g., to donate large sums of money, were obliged to go to said mother house, where, regardless of age or infirmity expected to participate in the life of the house.

Scrubbing floors until she was hospitalised did not appear to soften the heart of one elderly 'philanthropist' who did her best to alienate all other supporters irrespective of the consequences to the challenged addicts in recovery. She was opposed to the "American" Homeopath.

In this she was aided and abetted by the local GPs who told my patients that their complete cure of Hepatitis C was a 'Knock Miracle.' His associates, fans and admirers started a smear campaign against Homeopathy, to the effect that it was witchcraft, and not compatible with Catholic teaching.

Good thing they didn't mention that to Saint Mother Teresa of Kholkata/Calcutta!

The young men of the community walked miles back from the local GP's office to my home to tell me that they was no trace of Hepatitis C in their systems, that the local GP said it was a miracle, and intended to present it to the Vatican as such, but that they knew it was my work.

There is no Knock Shrine in New York and yet the same results prevailed there too. *However, I believe that all healing comes from the Creator, and the system of Homeopathy while precise, methodical, and belonging to the highest order of Science, is **miraculous in its efficacy***.

I wonder if the laboratory proof of my work at Knock was indeed, registered in the Vatican as a bona fide 'miracle,' because, by a strange 'coincidence,' my New York patients enjoyed the same success.

It would have saved many lives in Ireland were that laboratory proof published or noted – of course, keeping the names of the dear patients confidential.

I remember them with great affection and respect their struggle to regain and maintain sobriety.

Knock Shrine pays said doctor E50,000 per year to verify miracles.

It is likely that the Irish Government also paid him.

Further comment reserved.

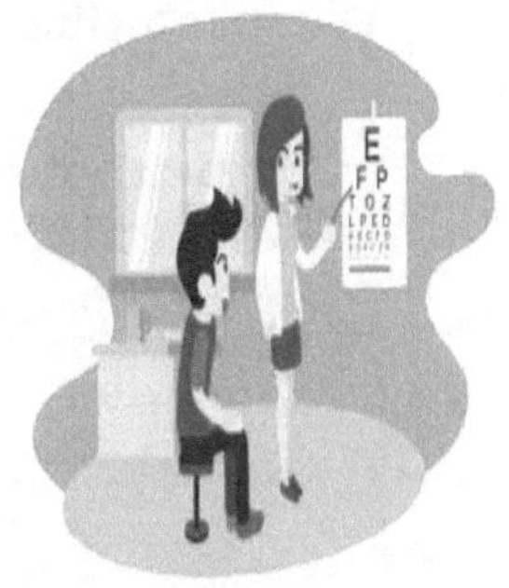

PERSONA NON GRATA – for saving a young man's sight! (Ireland)

The leader of the rehab community claimed to be Croatian, as did his alleged second in command. This was, however, a lie. The second in command was not another Croatian, but they broke all the rules, coming to my house at 11 pm after a member of the community was taken to hospital – allegedly – looking for espresso coffee – and pain killers.

I told him Homeopathy didn't work that way – and neither did their Community!

We do not mask or repress symptoms.

We prescribe according to the *totality of symptoms* and treat the **root cause** of the problem.

Once that is resolved, the associated pain 'melts away.'

I was also acutely aware that they were addicts *in recovery* – without benefit of AA, NA, etc., programs which I highly recommend. I was concerned that they were off the wagon and looking for drugs. Their frequent visits to the DVD Rental store for violent movies, proscribed by the Founders of the community was one cause for concern. Adrenal stimulants lead to anxiety lead to temptation to re-use, a perilous situation for them.

They were not pleased that I had no analgesics and I started to wonder how serious this particular group were about their recovery.

Their privileged position in Ireland was perfect for setting up networks.

Their testimony was pretty much the same – 'I hurt my parents, I'm sorry…'

Whereas the testimonials in AA and NA are deep, soul searching and diverse, each unique.

One system could certainly complement the other, but for some reason, Twelve Step programs were not allowed at the Community for recovering addicts.

On a subsequent visit to their Community, a young man, 'Ryan,' approached and asked to speak with me.

He explained that was having problems with his eyes, and when he described his symptoms I told him he needed immediate treatment, and I would arrange a consultation with an ophthalmologist whose skills I was assured of, or would treat him homeopathically if he preferred.

He chose the orthodox option.

It was a wise decision; with all the political harassment from NY and now Ireland, "follow ups"would be few and far between.   Besides Orthodoxy had our "Pilocarpus" and were using it – albeit more materially than us.

Medical standards vary widely in Ireland without any real controls. Even litigation is prohibitively expensive. An egocentric physician would be quite capable of dismissing the concerns of a Homeopathist in order to protect his own reputation or from downright prejudice or spite, so I felt it important to bring Ryan to a female opthalmologist that I trusted 100%, and who was kindly but lived in Clonmel some one hundred and fifty miles away.

I told Ryan that I would make arrangements for him to see the ophthalmologist, should he so wish, and that I was willing to pay for his treatment.

Ryan thanked me, and the gentle Tipperary Opthalmologist said that of course she would see him. A priest missionary friend generously agreed to drive him. *And then all Hell broke loose.*

The Croatian lads said that Ryan could not see the ophthalmologist because the other rehab 'houses' didn't have a Homeopathist. *They didn't have violent videos every Friday either!*

I asked if they were prepared to take responsibility for Ryan's complete and permanent loss of vision.

They still insisted that he could not see the ophthalmologist. There was some mention of the local GP, who habitually scoffs at my opinions, despite clear and unequivocal lab proof of Homeopathy's effectiveness, and who had apparently missed imminent danger to the young man's sight during his perfunctory *pro forma* screening of each candidate.

By God's grace there was a Youth 2000 conference in progress at the time, and the Spiritual Director of the Rehab House had returned from Peru for it. I approached him and asked why they were willing to allow a young man, 24 years young, to permanently lose his eyesight. Fr. Adrian was shocked and told me to tell them that Ryan was to see any physician that I chose and as soon as possible.

Ryan drove down a few days later with my dear Missionary friend, Fr. Martin, a Kiltegan priest, to Dr. 'Bernie' in Clonmel, where my suspicions of glaucoma were confirmed and his eyesight was saved. My friend in Clonmel, who refuses to be named, (but I've left a clue!) provided a prescription and report to the territorial local GP in the Knock area, and declined any payment for her service to the young man.

Due to the territorial 'sensitivities' of physicians in Ireland, Ryan's case was returned to the care of the local GP who continued to write the prescriptions recommended by Dr. Bernie and the young man's sight was saved.

I became suddenly *'persona non grata'* at the Rehab Community, and 12 out 15 members left in disgust at my exclusion, never to return.

I suspect that other abuses were going on, and wrote to the Religious Founders of the Community, who control from a distance but take no responsibility, despite demanding a high level of personal responsibility from their 'guests.'

Consequently, a system has evolved whereby letters to the Founders are intercepted and house leaders warned in advance.

The Founders may say that they 'didn't know' what was going on, and legally the young men are responsible for their 'houses.' However, the Founders decide who will be in charge, who gets moved around, and when and then step back to count the checks – or so it would seem.

The majority of the addicts in recovery are honourable; and subsequent leaders apologised to me, but the chinks in the armor need mending.

I also recommend that, at least 6 months before "graduation" that members attend 12 Step programs.

The Twelve Steps of AA

The relative success of the AA program seems to be due to the fact that an alcoholic who no longer drinks has an exceptional faculty for "reaching" and helping an uncontrolled drinker.

In simplest form, the AA program operates when a recovered alcoholic passes along the story of his or her own problem drinking, describes the sobriety he or she has found in AA, and invites people who are new to AA to join the informal Fellowship.

The heart of the suggested program of personal recovery is contained in Twelve Steps describing the experience of the earliest members of the Society:

1. We admitted we were powerless over alcohol—that our lives had become unmanageable.

2. Came to believe that a Power greater than ourselves could restore us to sanity.

3. Made a decision to turn our will and our lives over to the care of God AS WE UNDERSTOOD HIM.

4. Made a searching and fearless moral inventory of ourselves.

5. Admitted to God, to ourselves, and to another human being the exact nature of our wrongs.

6. Were entirely ready to have God remove all these defects of character.

7. Humbly asked Him to remove our shortcomings.

8. Made a list of all persons we had harmed, and became willing to make amends to them all.

9. Made direct amends to such people wherever possible, except when to do so would injure them or others.

10. Continued to take personal inventory and when we were wrong promptly admitted it.

11. Sought through prayer and meditation to improve our conscious contact with God AS WE UNDERSTOOD HIM, praying only for knowledge of His will for us and the power to carry that out.

12. Having had a spiritual awakening as the result of these steps, we tried to carry this message to alcoholics and to practice these principles in all our affairs.

People who are new to AA are not asked to accept or follow these Twelve Steps in their entirety if they feel unwilling or unable to do so.

They will usually be asked to keep an open mind, to attend meetings at which recovered alcoholics describe their personal experiences in achieving sobriety, and to read AA literature describing and interpreting the AA program.

AA members will usually emphasise to people who are new to AA that only problem drinkers themselves, individually, can determine whether or not they are in fact alcoholics.

At the same time, it will be pointed out that all available medical testimony indicates that alcoholism is a progressive illness, that it cannot be cured in the ordinary sense of the term, but that it can be arrested through total abstinence from alcohol in any form.

The best protocol for continuing recovery of any and every* form of addiction is regular attendance at AA or other similar, voluntary 12 Step programs combined with correct, expert, Homeopathic treatment to optimise recovery of organs and systems and to clear inherited markers from the suffering system.

*Exception for those "addicted" to criminal sexual activities.

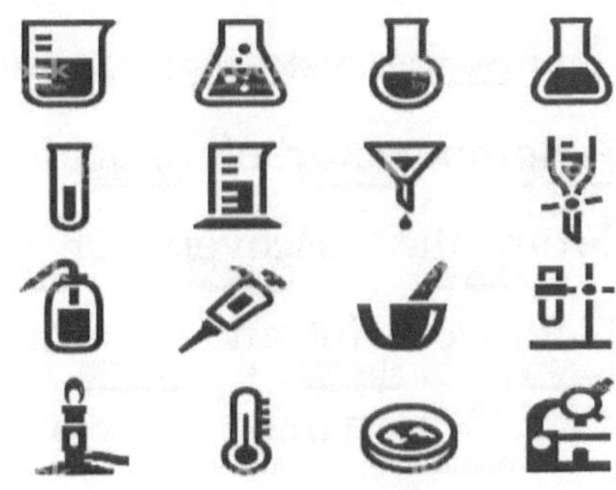

DR. NEMESIS

I have had the privilege of working alongside as well as for, some of the top specialists in the United States.

Mostly American born and raised, these men put their patients' welfare ahead of bigotry and ego. Egocentricity is too often the domain of the mediocre. In the arts as well as science, the greatest men and women are always the most gracious and humble.

If the others realised how many malpractice suits we could prevent, and have prevented, attitude to Homeopathy might change. Which is more powerful – Big Pharma or the Insurance Companies?

As is, however, authentic 'vocational' physicians do not have a problem with us; the battle is with Big Pharma who see profits plummet when patients are cured, whether by Homeopathy or 'unassisted miracles.'

To me, the system, inspiration and derivation of Homeopathy is nothing short of miraculous.

From the discovery of Cinchona (quinine) Bark by the Catholic Saint and Dominican friar, St. Martin de Porres of Peru, who named it for the Countess of Cinchon, a generous patron of his beloved poor, and sent it to Europe via the Society of Jesus, or Jesuits, to the 'Eureka' moment of the great Samuel Hahnemann who saw that in small quantities *it cured the same symptoms that it created in large quantities or 'material doses!'*

With 'ruthless' Teutonic thoroughness, Dr. Hahnemann embarked on a scientific journey of discovery which generated an *explosion* of imitative and inspired research and innovation, much of which is ongoing today as many of his insights and findings are pirated and plundered and which gave us the profound and meticulous Science of Homeopathy.

In addition to the extraordinary Materia Medica, Hahnemann gave us nutritional foundations for health, genetics, asepsis, environmental awareness, ie the importance of fresh and exercise, toxicology and more.

Sci-tech is still catching up with what Hahnemann called 'The Gift of our Gracious God.'

In fact, most of the positive developments in orthodox medicine have been ripped from the pages of the Homeopaths research.

Nothing 'New Age-y' there, my friends!

Would that orthodoxy had such Faith and Fidelity – we could work collegially for the betterment of humanity.

However, it is axiomatic that the more incompetent the physician – and there are some doozies out there – the more they will detest, despise and obstruct the work of the Homeopathist.

I fell foul of Dr. Nemesis, the Irish GP again, when I encountered a young man suffering a seizure on the floor of the Church.

The sacristan did not know what to do, and I did not have remedies on hand, but stood by to ensure that he did not injure himself.

In respect to the local 'territories,' and also because I believed the young man needed a CT or PET scan, I agreed that the worried sacristan should call the GP.

And so arrived Dr. Nemesis.

Angry at being called out – although it was his job for which, unlike me, he was well rewarded – he declared that the young man was drunk and that the Sacristan should call the police.

Now the young man had done no harm, had sought refuge and, apparently, healing, in the Church, and while the seizure had passed by the time Dr. Nemesis had arrived, the young man was still in a distressed state.

The police, aka, Gardai arrived, said 'ah, yes, this man is 'known' to us,' (a sure sign of guilt by Irish standards) and proceeded to pile him into their squad car.

I remonstrated, saying that he needed at least a EEC scan, but the Gardai rolled their eyes at Dr. Nemesis and said 'he's drunk!'

Even if that were so, alcohol toxicity can induce seizures and a tox screen should have been required before they dumped him in jail overnight.

I can attest to almost a dozen serious 'near misses' and misogynist abuse by said Dr. Nemesis who is paid by the local Church to prove and promote miracles.

In the meantime, he missed one rather spectacular one!

During the time that I spent in that area, the local Human Life International spent $16,000.00 to import a woman from the US, with no medical credentials whatsoever, to lecture and discredit all alternative medical systems competing with Big Pharma.

I could not fight this alongside superstition, venality, and such, and so limited my practice to established patients in the USA, and returned to writing.

I do, however, wonder how many lives would have been saved, had Dr, Nemesis had the integrity to send the lab reports re patients cured of Hep C to the appropriate Health Authorities in Ireland, and found one person with the courage to look further. This at a time when people were dying daily from Hep C contracted by transfusions with contaminated blood acquired from the USA.

There was a time when addicts sold their blood in and to hospitals in order to pay for the "next fix."

It is impossible to accept that they did not know the consequences.

THIS IS WHY HAHNEMANNIAN HOMEOPATHS MUST ANSWER ONLY TO OUR PEERS AND OUR PATIENTS. ALLOPATHY IS TOO ALIEN AND LIMITED FOR OUR REFINED AN EXACTING PROTOCOLS.

BROADWAY BLUES...

The concierge of one of NY's finest and most celebrated hotels called me one night and asked if I would consult with a guest. This is one of the hotels in NY where one can frequently spot Secret Service men outside in all weathers, risking their lives for a WH official or foreign dignitary.

I was relieved to find that the call was not on behalf of a UN delegate from a terrorist sponsoring nation but for a well-known and likeable Broadway Actress rehearsing for the opening night of a new show. We shall refer to her as 'BA.' Interpret anyway you like.

It quickly became clear that not only was 'BA' somewhat inebriated, but that she was not interested in a consultation, but a drunken phone therapy session - no fee expected. Her own salary was phenomenal. Not so likeable after all, then!

She was very agitated, anxious and upset, and knowing actors, I tried to calm her without getting into details about her relationship with her mom, or the day her plant died.

Not trivialising any occurrence in anyone's life – for example, the death of a neglected plant on the day that a beloved teacher or neglected grandparent dies can indeed trigger profound, reflexive issues of 'shame and blame,' but Miss BA was not interested in resolving her problems, only in dumping them at night, at what was, by that time, my private phone line.

I told her my fee for a house call – which was less than one night at her 'hostelry,' and given the late hour in NYC, and transport issues, more than reasonable – but she was not interested in providing professional respect or compensation; instead seemed to want a free therapy session on the phone which was not appropriate with a person whom I had never met, so I politely wished her well – as I do now – and hung up. My AA friends say, you cannot negotiate with a drunk.

I was, however, sad to see that she was fired from the show the following week.

Penny wise – pound foolish!

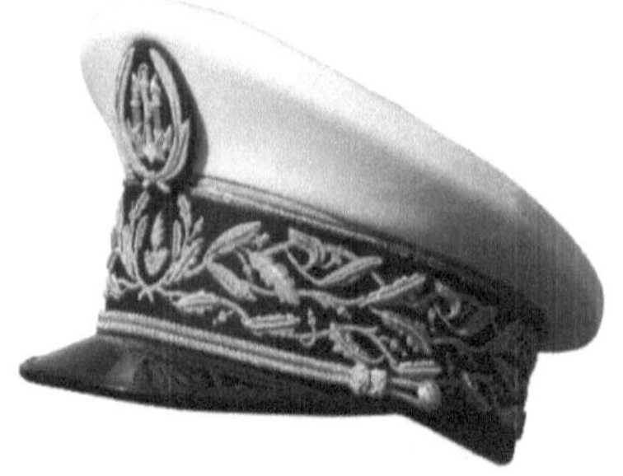

TREATING THE ENEMY – a WWII U Boat Commander! (Germany – NYC)

The daughter of a former U boat Commander, a German lady, 'Kay,' whom I greatly like and respect , asked me if I could 'do anything' for her father who suffered from Parkinson's Disease.

She told me, rather apologetically, that he used to lay mines along the English Channel, but quickly added that after the war he helped the British identify and remove them, and like many bona fide German military, detested Hitler and the Nazis.

Not enough to join the German Resistance – but then, already enlisted men hadn't a hope in hell of being demobbed or redeployed. Resistance meant death.

Sometime later she described the trek either near the end of WWII or just after, when they left their home near the seaport in Hamburg and took the long trail south to Berlin, for food. She spoke of the kindness of the British and the Americans to the German women and children, something she would never forget, she said.

She also did not "forget" the cruelty of the Soviets, who, in turn, were treated viciously by Stalin. Even up to the 1980s, defectors from Afghanistan stated at a Freedom House conference that they were forced to lick their Sergeants' boots clean. Just one of many abuses.

Back to the patient – 'Herr Commandant' was diagnosed with Parkinson's, detested the medication and seemed to be having abreactions and becoming rapidly worse.

I asked a few questions about 'Herr Commandant' diagnosed accordingly and two months later, Kay told me that 'Herr Commandant' no longer had Parkinsons, that the doctors believed they had misdiagnosed him, as he was walking about without any sign or symptom of Parkinsons whatsoever.

Thank God for Homeopathy!

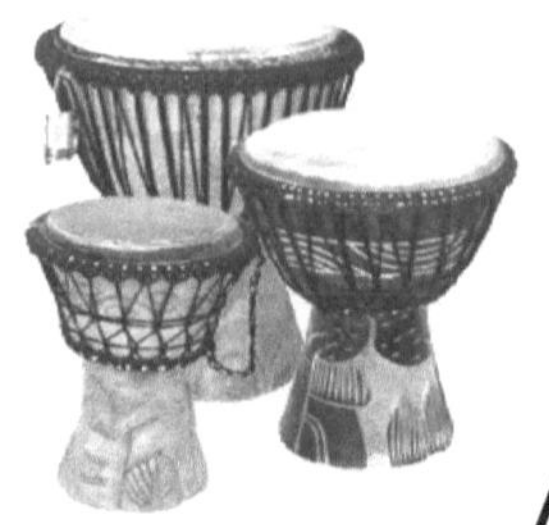

ANTHRAX AND THE AFRICAN DRUMMERS

Back in the mid noughties there was a small, contained outbreak of anthrax in NYC. It wasn't military grade and the victims were unlikely targets of then 'careful' jihadist groups, just students of African drumming, but it was a scare and a puzzle.

NYPD 'tecs went to work and found a lone teacher of African drumming and importer of *skins* which he processed himself in his Brooklyn loft.

A former neighbour, whose children attended his class, discovered that her children were experiencing respiratory distress, packed them off the hospital where they were diagnosed and treated.

One did not suffer from the respiratory systems but had a nasty looking 'eschar' - a black scar- by her ankle, which had persisted for days.

She turned to me for help. I made an exception to my 'registered patients only' rule as she was a fellow health professional asking for help for her child in distress, and so I treated the little girl.

The following day the eschar had disappeared and all but a faint pink tinge remained to tell of its existence.

I just wish I had taken before and after photographs.

Homeopathy can still surprise me with its rapid efficacy.

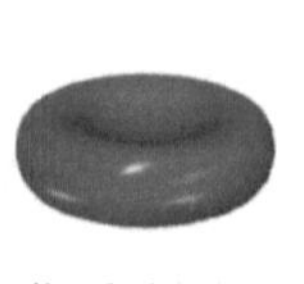
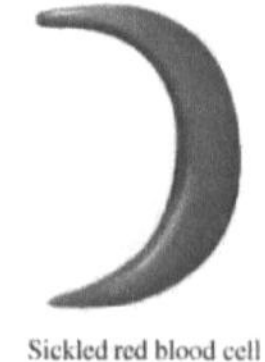

Normal red blood cell   Sickled red blood cell

RETINAL HAEMORRHAGE IN SICKLE CELL ANEMIA

One of the "eschar's" siblings, a teenager, suffered from Sickle Cell Anemia. One of the concomitants of the illness is periodic retinal haemorrhage, impairing vision and putting the victim at risk of permanent sight loss.

She was experiencing an acute episode when her mother asked:

'Could you do anything?'

One dose of the appropriate remedy, cleared the retina and the following day her vision was fully restored.

However, I was not invited to address other anomalies relevant to the brave teenager's condition.

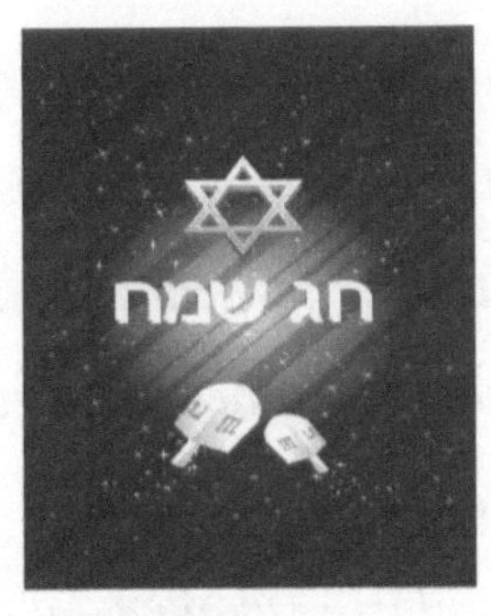

CHANNUKAH STORY – Torment and Triumph (Israel-NY)

One December morning, I received a call from a gentleman with a strong foreign accent. He wanted to make an appointment for his son.

His son was 42, he said and explained that his son was schizophrenic and that he would accompany him to my office, but remain outside in the waiting room during the interview.

His son was 'not dangerous,' he hastened to assure me.

I had no concerns. Schizophrenia has become a "generic" to cover a wide range of psychological issues and even symptoms of dietary deficiencies, not to mention misdiagnoses, prejudice and pure laziness.

In my experience 'schizophrenia' is an amorphous, ill- defined mental anomaly, used as a brick with which to bash political enemies, independent minded intellectuals, malnourished genius, wounded survivors of child sexual abuse, addicts riddled by STDs and other infections, Irish Catholics – particularly women, abused for ECT and other forms of research - and assorted other persons not willing to fit into pre- scribed boxes.

It was the last appointment of the day and he was late, but just as I started to prepare to leave, there was a gentle knock at the door.

I said 'Come in,' and went to open it just as an elderly man peeked in.

He seemed distressed so I offered him a cup of tea and invited him to sit down, an invitation which he accepted.

He apologised profusely for his son's absence, repeated that his son was schizophrenic and difficult. He identified himself as a Holocaust survivor.

I told him that at Yad Vashem I learned that the children of Holocaust survivors had greater difficulty dealing with their parents' suffering than the survivors themselves.

It surprised and puzzled researchers and psychologists, or so our guide had stated.

He was surprised that I had been to Yad Vashem.

I'll call my guest Yacov, after an uncle in law who is named on Schindler's List.

There was a long pause, one of many during that afternoon. Then Yacov started to speak of his childhood in Poland.

He spoke of his mother and father, of his sister and brother, none of whom survived.

'We were happy,' he said, describing the lighting of the Shabbas candles, the friends who would come around and pray, the bright oil lamps, the food, the *abundance* of food, the prayers, the laughter, the music, the sharing…

He spoke about Channukah, the nine days of gifts, of celebration, of visits and visitors, of the special foods and their historic and sacred symbolism.

I do not recall their occupations, but the impression of his parents was one of educated, cultured people.

And the day the Nazis came and dragged them off.

He described the horror, the filth, stench, hunger, cruelty, sadism, abuse.

More pauses.

The death of his mother.

The murder of his father.

Silence.

We sat there, two strangers, tears rolling down our cheeks, in silence.

The horror and the sorrow were overwhelming.

It seemed as if a minute and an hour elapsed before Yacov could speak again.

This time he spoke of escape.

How he and some other small boys managed to elude the guards during the processing of new prisoners, slip out and run for it.

He was all of seven years young at the time.

The Polish Resistance helped them, and by various means of transportation, they found themselves on a train to Switzerland.

He said that when they pulled into a station and saw Italian soldiers they ducked under the seats, but the Italian soldiers pretended not to see them, and that there was some difficulty at the Swiss border, but they were eventually admitted.

Here there is a 'concurrence.' Iwo Herzer's moving 'The Italian Refuge' describes an account by another refugee, of Jewish children spotting Italian soldiers running toward them and hiding under the seats as they halted at a station near the Italian-Swiss border.

The soldiers were throwing small, hard objects at them, but they were too frightened to look until the train started up again.

Imagine the surprise of those poor children when they saw that the 'missiles' thrown at them were actually – candy!!! Sweets! Caramelli! They had not seen sweets in years!

Ah, yes, 'the humanity of the Italians' of which Hitler complained in an irate telegram to General von Weisenheimer, his man in Rome. He was referring to Mussolini's covert sabotage of all attempts to deport Italian Jews.

I did not bring that up to Yacov. If he was one of those children, he was entitled to his memories, and if not, it would be too sad, another exclusion, another disappointment.

After the war he discovered that his siblings did not survive.

I left the questions aside, the 'research' questions – orphanage or foster care or kibbutz, or whatever.

They were, at that time, extraneous to occasion.

I just waited.

Yacov finished his tea, stood up and thanked me.

Tears were still rolling.

He asked what my fee was.

I said, 'no fee.'

He was surprised so when he offered again, I shook my head vehemently.

He shook my hand and said, 'thank you.'

I smiled and said,

'Shalom.'

He smiled, sunshine after the rain.

'Shalom,' he said, and left.

I never saw him again, but I hope he experienced some peace and love and recovery for his son.

For myself, I received a possible answer to the question at Yad Vashem where they said those who suffered intense bereavement and physical brutality at the hands of Hitler's cohorts, were better adjusted than their children?

I conjecture that they had *safe memories*. They had the experience, vital to a child's sense of safety and inviolability, of 'parental omnipotence,' a place to "go to" in the hell camps of Nazi Germany.

They also had a safe and happy world to 'return to,' at least mentally.

That world, as hard as they try to pass it onto their children, will require generations to repair, so that their children and grandchildren may *feel* 'safe' again.

I do believe Homeopathy would have helped both him and his son, if allowed, but for Jacov, the most essential, vital and immediate 'remedy' was Love.

"….and the greatest of these is the Gift of Love…" (St Paul of Tarsus)

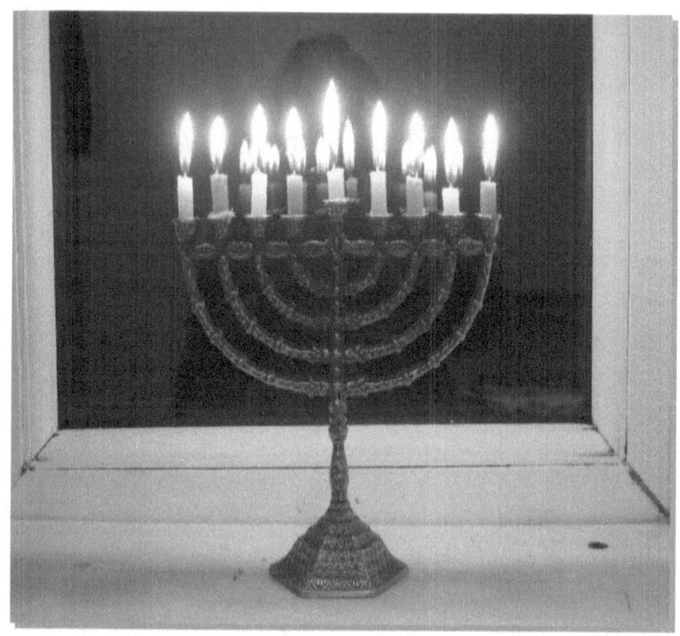

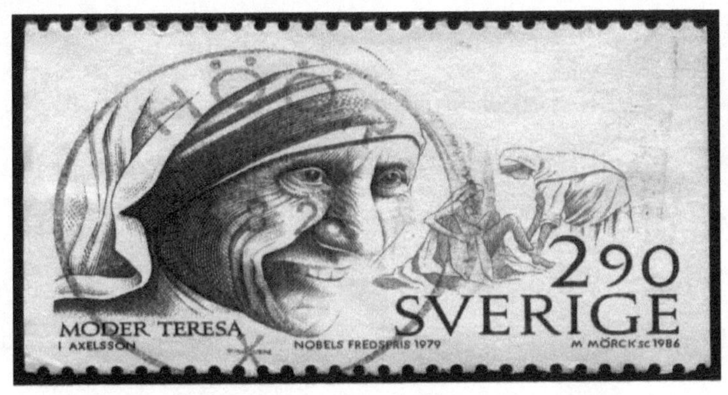

THE TINY, GREAT, SAINT TERESA of CALCUTTA India-NYC

There was considerable flak about Homeopathy which was gaining in strength in the USA in the eighties after a decade of one-on- one discussions with professionals in both the orthodox and alternative health fields.

The pharmaceutical industry with its 'dependency' medicine is a safe bet for investors – which is one powerful reason for the relentless assaults on the repeatedly proven effectiveness of Homeopathic Medicine.

Well, Big Pharma is a safe bet until one of the 'state of the art' 'double blind studies' is proven faulty and victims sue! Legal History and off-prime TV Advertising are full of such litigations.

'Double blind tests' are the stick used to abuse Homeopathy. We don't and won't do them. Besides they have led to one recall after another, and successive lawsuits related to horrendous injuries caused by FDA approved, double blind "proven" medications.

However, 'double blinds' are inappropriate for such a refined, precise, patient specific protocol as ours. Besides, the protocols established by the great Dr. Samuel Hahnemann, and embellished and illuminated by his followers, have stood the test of two centuries now. The only product 'recalled,' ie, confined to 'prescription use only' is Arnica tincture – and whoever caused that recall is a greedy, child hating - fill in your own - expletive.

Ironically, the only people allowed to prescribe Arnica are the very persons completely ignorant as to its use, power and limitation, ie, the MD in thrall to Big Pharma.

That being said – we face another challenge with frauds and cheats. Just as Orthodoxy has its incompetents, we have to deal with **pseudo** Homeopathists 'reading symptoms off blue tubes;' prescribing on the basis of one symptom; prescribing multiple remedies – MD 'fashionable converts' are the worst for that – and so on.

However, sincere, patient committed MDs become outstanding Homeopathists.

In my files is a prescription made by a Park Avenue MD/pseudo-'Homeopathist.' She prescribed 15 *high potency* remedies, *per day*…for one patient.

I can only conjecture that she started to ab-use Homeopathic remedies in order to avoid killing off patients with Orthodox medicine and her incompetence.

She guaranteed, however, that some patients would never recover…even under the care of a *bona fide* Hahnemannian Homeopathist, because by the time they found is it was to express regret that they had trusted orthodoxy.

They were too discouraged, defeated, butchered and broken to try our protocols despite expressing trust and saying they "wished (they) had come to us first."

Which is why, when I encounter someone who says they 'tried Homeopathy and it didn't work,' I ask a few questions re protocol and treatment, and then can honestly tell him/her - 'you did *not* try **Homeopathy**.'

Radionics and Homeopathy

I'll give radionics its own paragraph, as my mentor, Lionel Roy Ogden of Cambridge, England, practised radionics and introduced me to Homeopathy.

He did know his Materia Medica, and used a radionic block to expedite remedy selection for the suffering people crowding his waiting room.

I won't use that method.

I made an error by believing Carl Jung (I was 'jung' at the time) when he said that the picking of cards was not occultism but a resonance with the unconscious mind. (Memories, Reflections, Dreams) Of course when he wrote about entering his house and finding it choking with 'spirits' I should have run a mile.

Whether radionics is occultic, or whether a reflection of the unconscious, it bypasses the incredible teaching power of Homeopathy. The search for the precise remedy and potency provides profound insight into the integrative nature of the human body; into the complexity of plant, animal and mineral life, and the complexity of its effect on the human body; into constitutional uniqueness; into heredity; the power of the body to repair itself and to the reality of our co-existence on this earth. Every organism, every mineral, every atom on this planet has been subjected to the same forces and stresses as the human person, and IMO, there is a unique *sympathy* between them and us, a *sympathy provided and used by our "Gracious God" to heal and strengthen us.*

Because of radionics, however, many Christians cast a dim eye on Homeopathy, believing it to be superstition, occultism and worse.

For this reason, I wrote to Mother Teresa, knowing that in India she would have encountered *bona fide* Homeopathists. In fact, an Indian Minister for Health, a Dr. Kumar, had invited me to India in the seventies.

About two months after I wrote this letter, there was a tap on the door of my office. I opened it and to my surprise and delight, two Missionaries of Charity were standing outside.

Naturally I invited them in – Sr. Sylvia and Sr. Priscilla, two of Saint Mother Teresa's closest associates.

They invited me to assist their Missionary sisters in a Homeopathic capacity.

Naturally, I was delighted and found my life enriched and enhanced by the gentle Missionaries of Charity.

Some years later, as I was preparing to leave New York City, I emptied a book case and an envelope fell out.

It was addressed to Mother Teresa of Calcutta.

The letter had not been sent, and yet Blessed Mother Teresa of Calcutta had replied to it!

She and her sisters opened many Homeopathic clinics for her beloved poor.

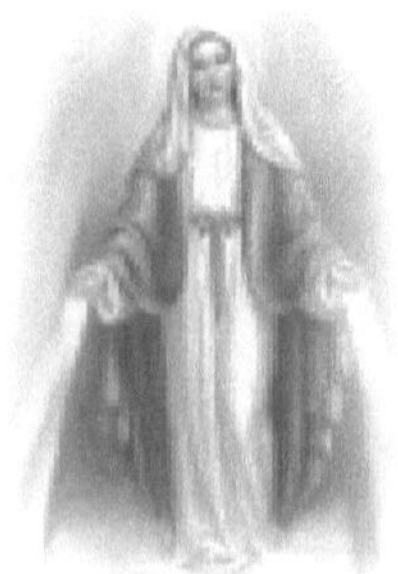 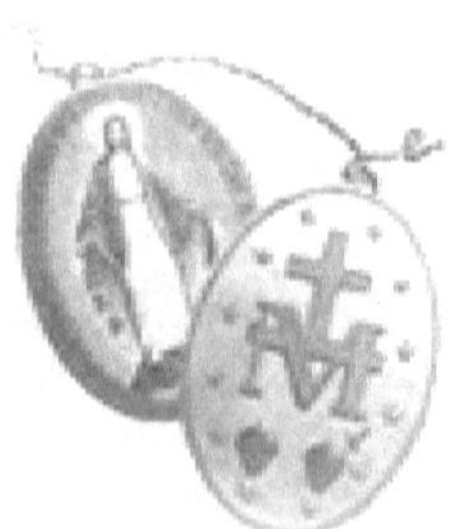 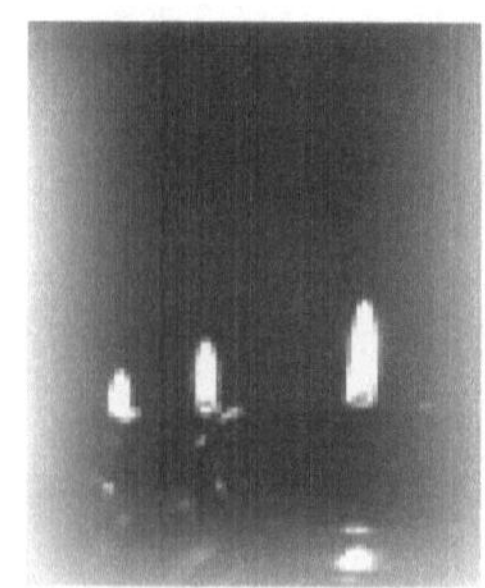

MEETING A SAINT

As I had consulted with the Missionaries of Charity, I was invited to meet Mother Teresa, now Blessed Teresa of Calcutta after a Mass for her sisters.

This was in Washington Heights, but I managed to find my way and work through the crowds surrounding the Church.

Because I was late, due to poor navigation on my part, I missed the group going directly to the Rectory via the Sacristy and had to go outside afterward, onto the street and back through more crowds into the Rectory. The MC sister who opened the door, recognised me and squeezed me through a tiny aperture.

The late, great John Cardinal O'Connor was leaving as I entered and gave me one of his warm smiles.

I was then ushered into a small room along with M. Teresa's ophthalmologist – who had removed a cataract from one eye – and his family, and waited.

The late British journalist and convert, Malcolm Muggeridge, who introduced Blessed Teresa to the West, described filming her. His crew said that it was too dark, and the film would not 'take,' but that when she entered the room it was as if the lights went on.

When Mother Teresa entered the small ante room where I was waiting, the lights were already on – but when she walked in, *it was as if they had been turned up to a higher wattage!*

A tiny figure appeared accompanied by the late Sr. Sylvia entered and the room became suddenly brighter.

Sr. Sylvia introduced me and M. Teresa took my hand, placed a handful of Miraculous Medals into it and said 'Come and See me in Calcutta.'

She then placed her hand on my forehead. The rest deserves a chapter to itself.

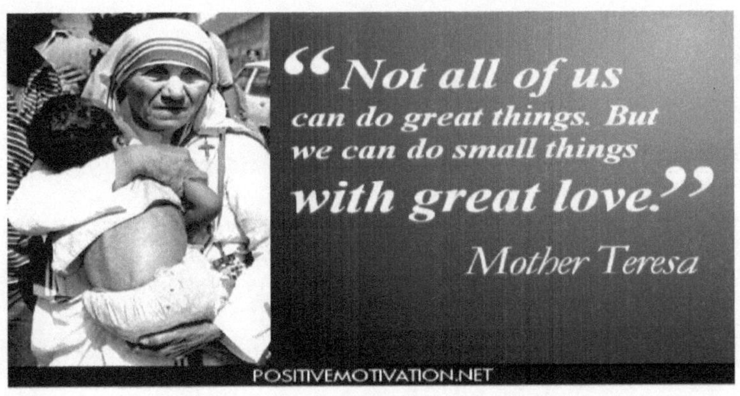

THE HEALING TOUCH OF MOTHER TERESA -

THE FIRST GOOD FRIDAY AGREEMENT

When Mother Teresa touched my forehead, it was as if the floor, walls, and ceiling had melted away and I was 'standing' in the middle of eternity, in a dark but peaceful night.

I 'blinked' back to the present, but she had continued on to her ophthalmologist and his wife, also waiting for her. Sr Sylvia smiled over her shoulder. She was so warm and kindly. I did not realise that was the last time I would see her. She died in a car accident along with another of Mother's 'Saints,' Sister Kateri.

I waited for Mother Teresa to leave the room, made my farewells and left the building. As I exited the main door of the Church, I saw hundreds of religious and laity amassed outside and felt a strange sense of 'usurpation.' They were all so much more worthy of the meeting than I - until I realised that 'worthiness' had nothing to do with it. The reason became clearer a month later.

However on those steps I felt a strong surge of love for the people outside, and started to hand out the Miraculous Medals earmarked for friends and family posterity!

I had, for a number of reasons, developed a phobia about flying. A few months after meeting Blessed Teresa, my brother invited me to his wedding in Spain. I reluctantly declined, but another family member insisted that I went, and bought tix on British Airways, knowing I trusted and once even enjoyed flying BA.

It was both a solace and exacerbation of my chronic homesickness for England. Yes, I know my fellow Homeopaths are 'screaming' the name of certain 'homesickness' remedies at me, and readers not raised in proto-terrorist 'cells' are – logically- thinking 'why not just go back,' but that's for another book.

At that time, too, Homeopathic remedies were not so easily available in New York City.

Well, the flight was booked for Good Friday! Penitential enough for the day, I thought, all factors considered. British Airways were kind enough to give us an upgrade to Business, which has forever spoiled economy class for me.

It being Good Friday, I requested a fish or vegetarian meal for myself, but on boarding was advised by Philip, named for one of Christ's Fishermen, that because of the special meal I could not avail of the upgrade.

The other family member said she would go back to economy as I was afraid of flying, and I said no, this was a big treat for her, and she said, well that was OK, so as we were debating who would enjoy Business Class on Good Friday, as other passengers struggled by, Philip rolled his eyes, went to the Purser and returned with assurances that we could both stay in Business Class and I would still get my piscine repast.

Later, as he served it, he advised me that they would bring me aloft to the cockpit after dinner.

Well it was a childhood dream to sit in the cockpit of a 747 in flight, but, but, but... I was now terrified at the mere idea, but still too committed to English 'good manners' to decline and follow my better instinct to hide under the seat!

After dinner when the lights were dimmed, Philip arrived with a lady crew member and a glass of champagne which they said to knock back, and they both directed me up the stairs and into the cockpit, where 'our chaps' - my childhood heroes, jolly English aviators, were cracking jokes about 'bumpy landings' and I literally felt like screaming and fainting at the same time.

Outside was just clear black starless sky, above, below, around, a cosmic emptiness interrupted only by the steady blinking of a line of lights crossing the Atlantic from New York to Europe.

I wanted to flee but was paralysed with fear. Bizarrely, the beauty of the scene was extraordinary.

Suddenly I was back in the room with Mother Teresa's hand on my head, and the sensation of the walls, floor and ceiling melting into eternity. A welcome peace came over me, even though physiological effects of 'jelly legs' remained, and I started to enjoy the silly jokes and the company of the successors of our great courageous RAF 'chaps.' We lost 14 every week during WWII.

Phillip returned to bring me back downstairs on my shaky 'pins' and the cabin suddenly looked like a large and comfy living room.

Later I had occasion to chat with Phillip in the galley.

 When I told him that I believed my phobia was rooted in contact with some of my late father's associates, proto terrorists training in the Middle East, he continued food preparation for a moment, then suddenly froze for a moment.

He then asked me to repeat what I had said and when I did so, he told me he was a Protestant from Northern Ireland. *Like many Protestants and Catholics in Northern Ireland he had lost friends in the extreme violence perpetrated by the Provisional, pseudo, IRA.*

We shook hands and remained friends for the rest of the flight.

That was the day of the Good Friday Agreement when the IRA agreed to lay down their arms – in return for money, rights and privileges.

'Casualties' of the conflict, such as myself, with my invisible wounds, and, indirectly, Philip and others North and South of the border, were tossed aside for political expedience.

But I have flown thousands and thousands of miles since then with minimal apprehension. *Thank you, Mother Teresa!*

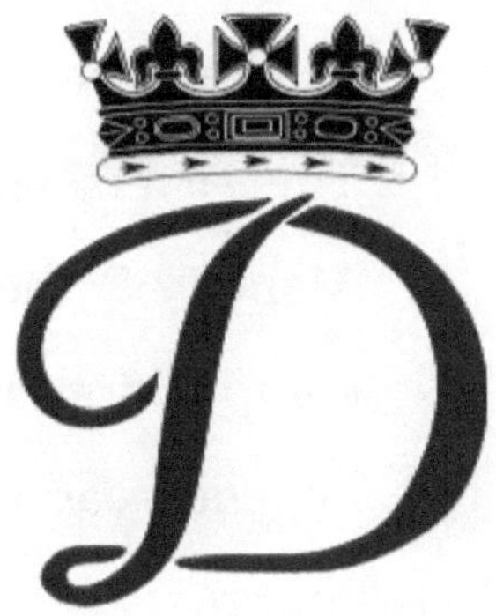

MOTHER TERESA and the ENGLISH PRINCESS (England – NYC – India)

I had the opportunity to meet the late, sweet, Princess Diana, and did not 'seize it with both hands.'

Had I known that the following week her dying words, 'my boys, my boys,' would be splashed on headlines around the world I might have taken the opportunity.

The dear Sisters, Missionaries of Charity shared her last visit with me. They said 'Princess Diana was *like a daughter* to Mother Teresa.'

Their chapel is bare, spotless and beautiful. There is a large crucifix with the words 'I Thirst' above the image of Jesus, and a statue of the Virgin Mary.

There are a few chairs for visitors or the disabled and elderly sisters.

The sisters sit on the floor during Mass and prayers. Many of their hymns are original both in music composition and in lyrics. When they sing, they sound angelic – as one would imagine a chorus of angels to sound.

When Princess Diana arrived, the sisters brought her into the chapel to wait for Mother Teresa. They brought a chair for her, placed it in the center of the chapel floor and sat around her, singing.

They gave her a foretaste of Heaven.

When Mother Teresa came downstairs, the sisters left, and they spoke for almost two hours.

Princess Diana was 'radiant' when she left Mother Teresa. After her death, a few short weeks later, a cartoonist depicted them walking up to Heaven hand in hand.

It was a sweet and consoling image for two sweet and consoling women, each a "queen of hearts" in her own domain.

"They have gone ahead to prepare a place for us..." wrote Saint Mother Teresa in a note of condolence to me.

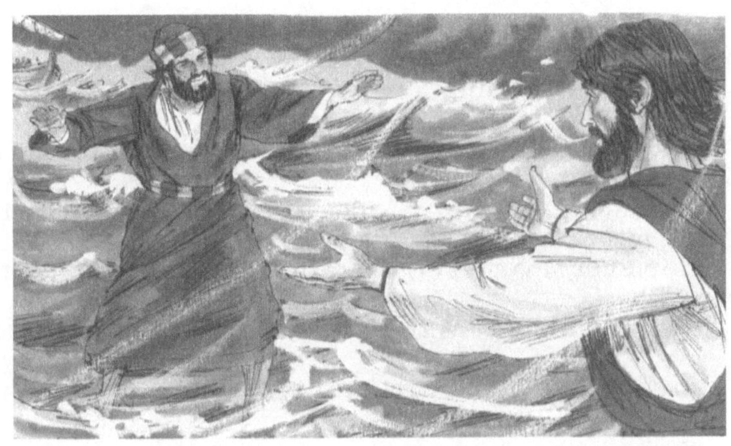

ISRAEL – STILL A LAND OF MIRACLES

My work brought me into contact with persons with disabilities, some still active in the work force, some, volunteering; others just getting by.

It helped me understand the difficulties of manouevring a wheel chair through NYC, getting up and down subway steps on crutches and wheeling rubber tires across acres of carpet in well- meaning but ill-advised hotels.

It led me to write about this in various news outlets for the disabled, and subsequently to Israel.

As a result of the many wars and acts of terror waged against Israelis in the last sixty plus years, Israel has a significant population of disabled soldiers and citizens. Added to the exigency is the antiquity of the cobbled streets, and the hilly slopes of some cities, e.g., Jerusalem. However, every consideration has been made for chair users; while we were in the throes of the ADA act, Israel already had basic cuts and ramps at sidewalk crossings, etc.

Homeopathic remedies were available there too.

Which was just as well for a young, very attractive German TV journalist, 'Greta,' working for a French TV station and doing a story on Israel.

Our guide was a Berber, a former commando who guided the IDF members through the desert.

When I met Greta, her fair skin was red and blistered from the hot sun and desert treks. She was in considerable pain and discomfort.

Aloe used topically, brought her considerable relief, but it was the 'internal' Homeopathic potential (aka remedy) that astonished everyone.

The following morning, the blisters had disappeared, and her skin a pale pink, with barely any tenderness.

The Berber begged for the name of the remedy, but I did not tell him.   I would prefer to give a course on Homeopathy than to provide the name of *one* remedy that might not be suitable for the next patient, and would be used indiscriminately, then throw Homeopathy into disrepute, and the "we tried Homeopathy and it didn't work..." comments from persons who read a symptom from a blue tube.

On a different case, a different remedy might have been more appropriate.   Homeopathy is too precise for 'one size fits all' prescriptions.

That being said, I used the same remedy for one of Mother Teresa's volunteers, a supermarket manager, who sustained a *chemical* burn to his eye from a splash of lye, and was in considerable pain, discomfort and blurred and painful vision for several days.

The following morning he called to thank me and say that his pain was completely gone and his vision was fully restored.

Small miracles in Israel – for example, the threat of a rain storm almost forced the guide to cancel the trip on Lake Kenneret (Gallilee).

I suggested we "ask the Prophet Elisha'"to hold off the rain, and he did – until the guide started talking about Baptists jumping into the lake in the middle of thunderstorms. One of our group members said it would be exciting to see a storm and imagine Jesus walking on the water toward St. Peter, and suddenly lightning pierced the sky, and a storm broke.

It lasted a few minutes, but delighted the pilgrims and writers present!

Another 'small' miracle happened along the Via Dolorosa. I was making a photo record of the Stations of the Cross, most of which were marked.

The Ninth Station however, where 'Jesus meets the Women of Jerusalem' took place where the cobbled roadway intersects with a market place and posted no signs.

"I'll photograph it anyway," I thought, raising my camera – *just as a flock of white veiled young women of Jerusalem 'appeared from nowhere'* and stood in front of it!

As G.K. Chesterton once wrote: *'To those who have Faith, no explanation is necessary, but to those who have none, then no explanation is possible!'*

Again, in the desert on Mother's Day, sitting on a rock, feeling rather blue and guilty for not being with my teenagers – presumably piling up used dishes and pizza boxes pending my return – I was delighted when a partridge suddenly appeared out of nowhere, a mother hen followed by her five chicks. They walked toward me and I remained very still as they passed closely by me and disappeared again.

It was as if God patted me on the shoulder and said, 'it's OK, 'Mom,' you'll see your chicks again…'

I do not know who, in the Israeli Ministry of Tourism, or El Al, made the arrangement, but I am eternally grateful for the First Class upgrade on the return flight.

'Welcome Home' said the immigration officer at the JFK El Al Terminal as I bounced off the long flight, so tanned and fit that my neighbors didn't recognise me!

And yes, the emptied pizza boxes and pile of dishes awaited me. I took it as a compliment. Like cats, they found a way to say they missed me…

'Welcome Home' indeed!

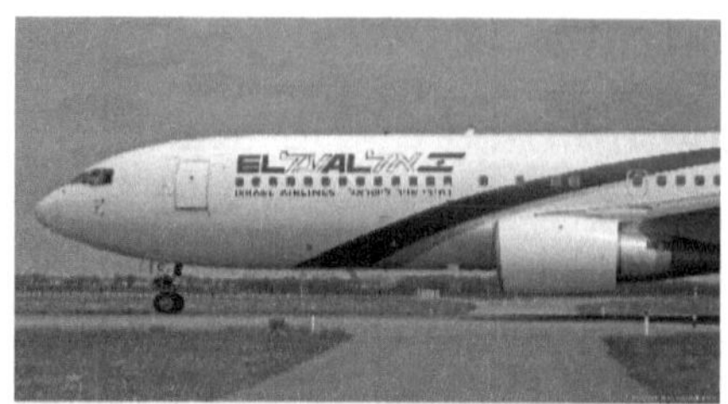

MIRACLE?   COINCIDENCE? – "MYSTEROUS WAYS..."

My visit to Israel has some bearing on the second visit of the Holy Father, Pope John Paul II to New York City.As guests of El Al Airlines and the Israeli Tourist Board, I and a group of writers were invited to observe 'routine maintenance' on one of their 747s.

Every three years, their jets are gutted and re-assembled thread by thread, screw by screw, wire by wire, every single item counted and accounted for.

One of the mechanical engineers was a Russian wearing a Guinness t-shirt!

As I was invited by reason of my interest in and work with persons with disabilities, the El Al execs took great pride in showing me their 'ElAlift.'

It was years ago, so I'm not sure if the spelling is correct. It's probably standard now, but it was unusual then, a lift using a 'scissors' fulcrum to bring wheelchair users from the ground to the boarding area.

Shortly after my return, I bumped into Cardinal O'Connor's Secretary, a gentle Monsignor with an eidetic memory and a huge heart who is now an Archbishop, an Archbishop who came from the pomp and circumstances of his Episcopal Ordination in Rome to a public hospital ward to administer last Sacraments to a prostitute dying of AIDs. Wow!

At the time of our encounter, everyone was asking for the return of John Paul II, so I took advantage of the meeting to ascertain if, and when, John Paul II might visit New York City again.

Monsignor shook his head sadly, and mentioned that since the attempt on John Paul's life, he was unable to climb the steps required to ascend to a platform where he would be visible to all.

"What about an El Alalift?" I asked, not ready to give up.

"El Alalift?" he asked quizzically.

I was sure he had places to go, people to see, but this kindly man never, ever, gave the impression that there was any other person in the world but the party that he was addressing.

I explained El Alalift to him, and he listened carefully.

I hope El Al doesn't mind too much, but I also suggested that they might lend him one.

He thanked me and went on his way.

A short while thereafter, it was GAME ON!

Announcements were made, and dates were set.

The Holy Father, John Paul II, was on his way!

Whether or not El Al's own lift was used, but it was inspirational, and also facilitated the great late Pontiff's access to many of the altars on which Mass was offered.

Whether or not the confluence of circumstances was coincidental or a 'succession of small miracles' is debatable.

However, as GK Chesterton once wrote: *To those who have Faith no explanation is necessary, to those who have not, no explanation is possible!*

Or, as scripture puts it 'His eye is on the sparrow...'

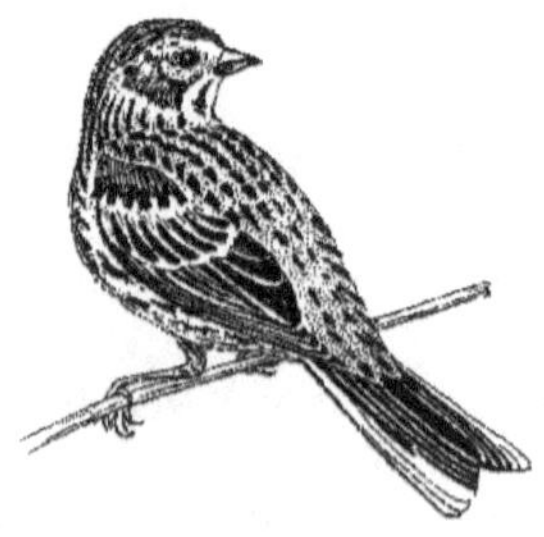

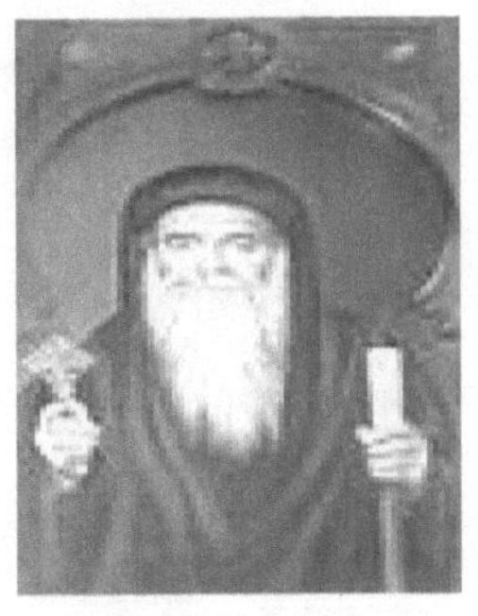

COPTIC MONSIGNOR (Egypt – NYC)

This heroic man (not pictured) eventually became a registered patient, but I first encountered him in the Respiratory Unit of a municipal hospital in New York, visiting him at the request of the chaplain, the late, much missed Timothy Healy, SJ.

He was in agony; hemiplegic - one side paralysed after a stroke, fed by a stoma, or tube, surgically inserted into his stomach, attached to a respirator and subject to constant infection. Furthermore, he shared a room with at least three other patients, some of whom were more alert than he and had no compunction about turning the volume on their boom boxes (CD/radios) to intolerable levels. Life before MP3/4s!

He had endured this for eighteen months!

In addition to which, as I discovered later, one or two members of the nursing staff made his life miserable once they understood that he was a Catholic priest.

Had these racists understood that he was a Coptic Rite Bishop of Egyptian Birth and Turkish heritage, they may have controlled their Christophobia. An element of anti-white racism permeated the municipal hospitals that I knew well; the local politicians kept an eye on grass roots public jobs and stacked them accordingly.

I started to visit him regularly; at one point discovering him in a separate room stretched out as if on a cross, and surrounded by medical personnel –'centurions' trying to stick nails, ie, needles into his feet and hands in an effort to located an undamaged vein.

He had chronic infections, a result of the treatment rather than the illness, and, from observation, I was certain that I could help him.

After discussion with the Director of Respiratory Medicine, the Provincial of the Order, and his 'Next of Kin' who was also an MD, and the Archdiocese to whom he had been seconded, and of course, the Coptic Monsignor himself, it was agreed that I start treatment.

One week later he was free of infection. A month later, on room air, i.e, off respirator all day, until evening time.

Two months later he was wheeling himself about the hospital, concelebrating Mass and one month after that, he was down again.

His brother had persuaded him to undergo the implantation of a Diaphragmatic pacemaker, still in development/experimental stage, and so after two months of freedom, the dear man was under the knife. The rationale being that the Med Director was understandably cautious about the risk of sleep apnoea. Then again, despite his professional affirmation of my work, he didn't really know just how much a Hahnemannian Homeopathist can do for a multiply compromised patient.

I was certain that had he remained exclusively under Homeopathic treatment, that he would eventually have left the hospital and returned to his mother house, but I realised that the orthodox physicians were highly conscientious and did not know enough about Hahnemannian Homeopathy's spectacular results to trust us completely.

Despite the compelling evidence before their eyes. And so my unspoken fear that he would not return to active duty at his Provincial House was fulfilled.

With Homeopathy's help, however, he recovered quickly enough from the surgery without further infection. I did, however, have to intervene when he became comatose.

Soon enough, he was moved from the Respirator Unit to the Nursing Home Unit at a saving to his Insurance provider of $1,000 **per day.**

Without Homeopathy, this would not have been possible.

While my dear friend did not permanently leave the hospital, he subsequently enjoyed many visits to his Provincial House, to his Coptic Church and to the Holy Father, John Paul II's Masses.

The Administration, once apprised that such an erudite gentleman was in their Nursing Home unit, provided him with a large single room overlooking the river, where he became a valued and beloved volunteer auxiliary chaplain for his remaining years, on call 24/7 to staff, visitors and his fellow patients and residents.

Coincidentally he had attended seminary in Lyons, France, which has a world renowned Homeopathic Pharmacy. If his 'Cause' goes forward I'd like to 'claim' him as the Patron Saint of Homeopaths!

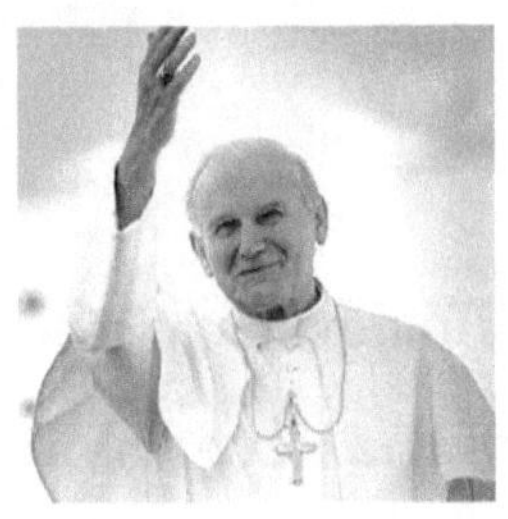

THE COPTIC MONSIGNOR AND THE HOLY FATHER JOHN PAUL II. (NYC-Rome-Egypt)

At the Aqueduct Raceway, five husky Franciscan friars carried Monsignor's wheelchair up five flights of steps to the platform where the priests would concelebrate the Sacred Mass with the Holy Father.

As we waited, a flock of doves rose and dived around a tree, moments before JPII's chopper arrived and landed on the ground outside the platform.

I stood up and looked over the side.

The Holy Father, John Paul II stepped out of the chopper and looked up directly at me.

I froze. There were no protocols for greeting a Pope at the private school of my English childhood.

'Should I curtsey?' I wondered, staring at the Holy Father.

His face broke into a megawatt smile, and he waved, and I waved and that smile is forever in my heart.

Central Park

I did not need the husky friars to take Monsignor to the Central Park Mass, but they were there, helpful as ever, and afterward we enjoyed the hospitality of none other than the Grand Duke of Austria and his beautiful, American wife, Elisabeth!

One of Geza von Hapsburg's forebears was the great saint, Princess Elizabeth of Hungary, whose services to the poor and Franciscan generosity and simplicity are legend. He and his wife are gentle, kind, hospitable souls.

The young friars had spent the previous night sleeping on the floor of their Lexington Avenue apartment – large by New York standards, but not sufficient for half a monastery!

I suspect that they offered to host them in a hotel, but the friars, true to their Franciscan spirituality, would decline that.

The Mass itself was interesting – concelebrating priests sidelined then Police Commissioner, William Bratton, sidelined, and outside the 'celebrity zone,' while what seemed to be the brashest stars on Broadway challenged the goodwill of the devout congregation sitting on grass, or uncomfortable folding chairs while waiting for the real star, John Paul II.

The Holy Father finally arrived to outstanding applause and relief!

He must have read our hearts, because, during an address to us, he suddenly broke out into a beautiful Polish Christmas Carol, in a strong, unaccompanied, a capella voice.

After that, everyone settled and the Mass continued with due reverence.

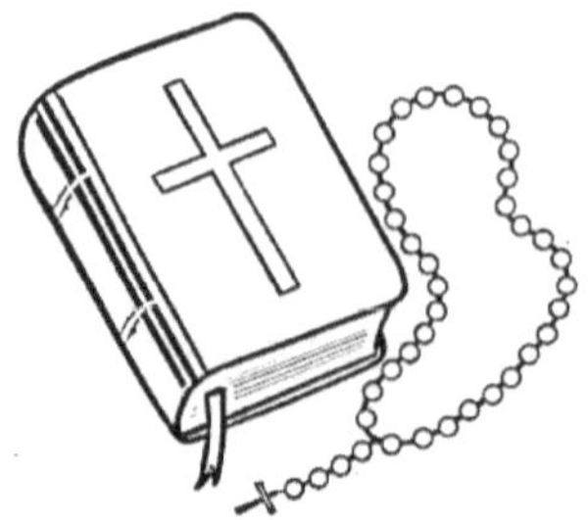

INDEFATIGABLE – HOORAY FOR HOMEOPATHY!

When I returned him to the hospital, seven hours after 'springing' from his ward, the indomitable Monsignor, who had to rise at five am and miss at least one 'in stoma' feed of Ensure for at least four hours, thanked me profusely and then said wistfully,

'I so wish I could attend the Rosary!'

'No more tickets, no special passes,' I replied, sad to disappoint him, but glad to 'put my feet up,' so to speak.

He must have had a 'hotline to Heaven,' because when I returned to my apartment there was a Special Delivery package from the Archdiocese of New York with... passes to the Rosary!

Hmmm

And so we went, again, up at 5 am, one feed for Monsignor in the morning, over the river, across the sidewalks, along the avenues of New York and through the police barricades surrounding St. Patrick's Cathedral.

And the previous year he'd been stretched out on the hospital bed for eighteen months, unable to speak or move any part of his right side; now he was wheeling his chair independently, sipping beef broth and diluted orange juice, blessing his friends, hearing confessions, speaking through a trach tube, breathing normally – except when they put him on a precautionary respirator at night.

I was hoping that Monsignor would have the opportunity to meet John Paul II, and I am certain that had I been able to apprise the late, great hearted Cardinal John J O'Connor that the Coptic Monsignor would attend the Holy Father's rosary, then Cardinal O'Connor would have arranged for him to be at the Sanctuary with his brother priests.

It was not meant to be. Or perhaps some overwhelmed usher 'got in God's way,' but it was still a delightful, prayer-filled and profound experience.

The same lovely Englishwoman, Anne, at the Archdiocesan Office of Disabilities, who sent the 'Hail Mary' tickets, had also provided tickets for two of my dearest, disabled patients.

To their delight, the Holy Father stopped by their pew and took their hands.

He didn't have to know their story. He read their hearts.

A hallmark of sanctity.

The staff at Goldwater Hospital deserve a gold medal award for going off routine in order to facilitate Monsignors 5am preparation and 6 am departures.

They had some bad apples, certainly, but the majority were dedicated and compassionate. Shining stars in the firmament of hope.

At last report the hospital was undergoing conversion into luxury apartments overlooking the East River and facing the UN. Patients were shipped to the suburbs and upstate; for many of them losing their home of many years, their "orientation" and their mates.

In revising and revisiting these moments, they seem mysteriously connected. My work with the disabled led to a visit to Israel, to the ElAl Lift, to the Papal visit, to Monsignor's "escape" from the hospial and the concelebration of Mass both at St. Patrick's Cathedral and in Central Park. "For those who have Faith, no explanation is necessary. For those without, none is possible." GK Chesterton.

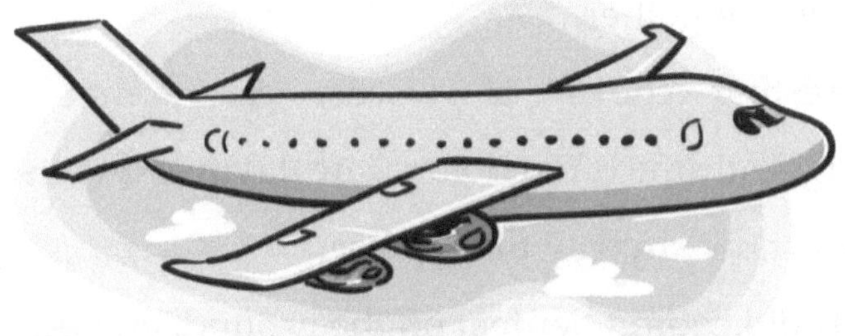

THE CASE OF THE AIRSICK AIR CREW

Vincit Omnia Amor!

Love conquers all? Not in the case of the air hostess and her pilot boyfriend.

A low fare special to Italy. The 'sardine can' effect. Maximum income for minimum outlay. Hundreds of holiday makers jammed into a small jet with one narrow aisle. The inevitable hustle to sell drinks and food…

…along with apologies for the delay in service.

One of the crew members was air-sick in the back of the plane; another crew member was helping her. This always happened at the beginning of the flight, but she was usually better by the end…

And why did she continue to fly?

Her boyfriend was the pilot and this way they could 'layover' together.

Interesting choice of words, given that particular 'budget' airline offered very few 'layovers' to its crews.

Did I know anyway to help her?

Short of keeping her feet on the ground, er, yes.

'See a Homeopath.'

'Is that herbs and stuff?'

'No, that's Homeopathy and science.'

'Are you one?'

'Yes.'

'Can you give her something?'

'I don't even know her…'

'I'll see if she'll come up to you…'

'That's ok. Is she fair, skinny and…?' I asked, not wanting to 'lead' her.

'No, she's fair and, not exactly plump, but…'

'Sitting down and a glass of water – would that help?'

'No, it's when she sits down for take-off it starts and the water just sets her off…'

Anything else? Anything unusual?

"She also gets car sick."

"So it's movement plus … confinement…"

"I'll ask her but she's in the bathroom getting sick…"

More out of compassion for the crews that had to double up while working for a less than kindly boss, I wrote 'See a professional Homeopathist about this,' and the name of the remedy that I considered appropriate on a card and gave it to the concerned friend of the air-sick, love-lorn stewardess.

No feedback, no thanks expected.

On a number of occasions I have helped other passengers by using acupressure points to temporarily relieve anxiety, particularly with smokers undergoing withdrawal symptoms.

There are Homeopathic remedies, but without a commitment it is a waste of time and energy to treat the casual and uninformed, unless the situation is acute or critical.

Chamomile herbal tea is helpful in such situations, but few airlines carry it, and few smokers of my acquaintance like it! A breakfast or light supper of oatmeal is also calming, and provides essential stamina to see passengers through today's stressful airports.

Persons with any form of anemia should board as late as is courteous and possible as 'clean air' standards have dropped considerably – offset on the other hand, by proscriptions on smoking, and the less time spent on board, the better.

Nothing works better and with a stronger opportunity for permanent recovery than Homeopathy, especially where the condition is Constitutional.

Caveat: While acute conditions respond rapidly, some say "miraculously" to the well-chosen remedy, chronic conditions often take a little bit longer, and require regular follow ups.

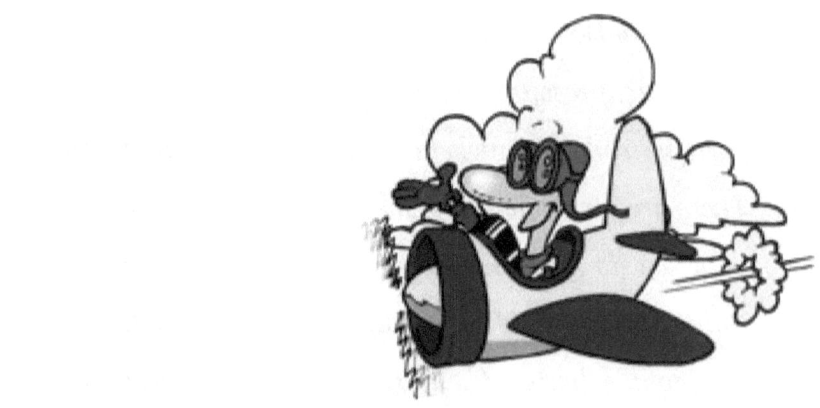

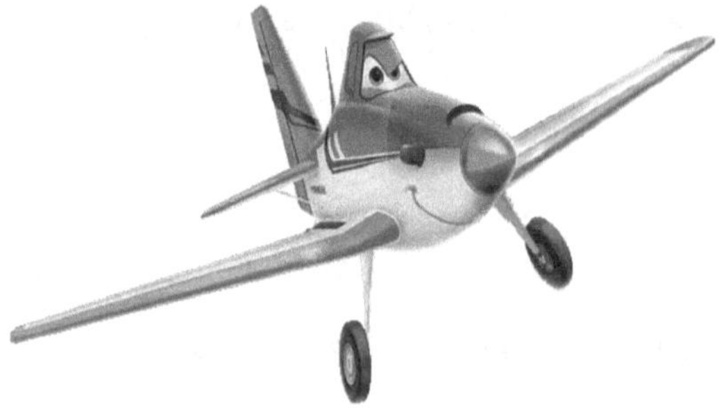

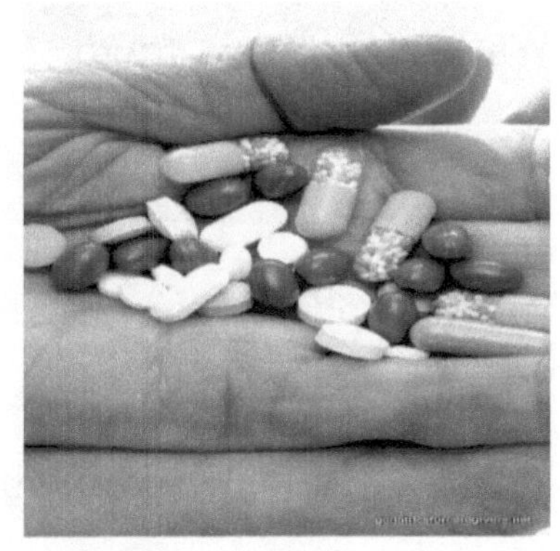

THE PARANOID PEDIATRICIAN

Another overseas excursion took me to Germany to a conference on Science, Religion and Philosophy.

We arrived at Munich Airport and were driven by luxury coach to a town in the foothills of the Bavarian Alps. It was stunningly beautiful, a cross between The Sound of Music and one of those scenes where allied soldiers come across a beautiful meadow, let down their guard until the greenswards turn red to the sound of machine gun fire.

The EU wants us not to 'mention the war,' but its shadow still looms over a coercively united Europe, where excess and absurd regulations keep people in a state of anxiety and suspense.

Most bizarre, of course, are proscriptions against classic, Hahnemannian Homeopathy.

Walking into town, we suddenly found ourselves approaching rail tracks and stopped in unison, standing speechless for a moment, then exchanging glances in frozen silence, collectively remembering The War – the movies, the news reports, the broken relatives.

At the time, we were all strangers.

Another reference to the war occurred when older women would approach like Panzer tanks and try to push me off the road. It was so frequent that the gallant men in the company would start to block them.

After two days of this, once the jet lag wore off I realised that my tiny British-American flag pin was probably evoking very painful memories, and so, reluctantly, I removed it.

My English childhood was happy, so the flag pin represented good cheer.

However younger Germans feel about the war and its postlude, it was clear that the elderly were still in pain.

As a later visit to Dachau showed, it took twelve years of bullying, assault, kidnapping, murder, smashed presses, 'disappearing people, etc., by an Austrian usurper, to turn the people of Germany into compliant, robotic Nazis.

Was my flag pin insensitive, or was it a form of self defence? I took a stop-over in London so that I could arrive in Munich on British Airways.

The truce may be signed and the elites go out and celebrate, but the people of lesser privilege, who clean up, rebuild, tend to the injured -'get on with it,'so to speak - carry their wounds, visible and invisible, to the end of their lives.

And, as with the innocents of Auschwitz, pass them on to their children.

As we sat down for a supper of processed meats, cheese, bread and coffee a harried looking man joined us.

He seemed intelligent and introduced himself as 'Ivan,' a paediatrician. He was not one of the Eastern Europeans at the conference, some of whom had different motivations for attending the conference.

As he did.

The following day, after a breakfast time imitation of the scatty White Rabbit in Alice in Wonderland, he confided to me that he had come to Germany to commit suicide.

Silence, any cynics out there! Even when hyper rational as in authentic OCD (Obsessive Compulsive Disorder) mental health issues are by definition, *irrational*.

Dr. Ivan spoke of his addiction to prescription drugs, supplied by his medical friends, and that he was 'on withdrawal' and would be happy to undergo Homeopathic treatment.

Oh yes? Oh no!

Talk about being between a rock and a hard place!

The 'enemy' had crossed camps and sought my help but at what a price!

Perhaps requesting my professional help was his insurance policy – to prevent me from going outside professional limits…to personally compromise me and my work.

He assured me that he had gone cold turkey, was undergoing withdrawal, and would accept my protocols.

I took him at his word. I mean, who wouldn't trust a paediatrician.

At least till I observed him ogling the body of an eight year old gymnast/circus entertainer in a leotard performing aerial lifts, etc., with a much older man, on the chilly streets of the Czech Republic.

Still in Germany I was very frustrated with the progress of Dr. Ivan. His face would brighten and vitality return within a few minutes of the 'well chosen' remedy, but every morning he arrived at the breakfast table, addled, 'hung over,' confused, muttering to himself…

…still denying use of narcotics, psycho-tropes, etc.

Hmmm

He had played a strong sympathy card. With his 'suicidal intentions' hanging over me like a sword of Damocles, I was reluctant to abandon him. He had become dependent on our evening walks, even as the other 'devout Catholics' started to gossip about an 'affair,' and asking who was the woman leading this good 'married man' astray, etc.

'Ivan's' grandfather supported Hitler, he said. His first wife committed suicide, leaving him with 10 kids to raise; she was schizophrenic, he said. He re-married, an ambitious woman with two young daughters, one five, one eight, and a redneck ex-husband with whom she was still 'friendly.'

He started to extol the beauty of the little girls in their 'marching band' outfits and their 'gymnastic outfits.'

Later, in Prague, I was to wonder if the little gymnast reminded him of his step daughters or if something else was on his mind.

Something he had to shut-down with pills, perhaps.

In Prague the musicians, street, church, whatever and wherever, were outstanding. The mechanical clock was amazing. The restaurants were full of duck: duck a l'orange, duck aux cerises, duck - and duck and duck...

The rivers weren't.

The hotel menu's choice of vegetable was: carrot, carrot, or carrot.

'Thank you, I'll have the carrot!'

Prague to me will be the eternal cold and damp and cold. I'm sure that it has developed beautifully since that long ago visit, but the memory of standing in damp, run down churches and walking slowly through the town squares chills me to the bone to this day.

It was late Spring, and as I expected to be staying exclusively in Bavaria, which is Southern Germany, I brought only a light jacket. The chill had started when we crossed into former East Germany and across the still bleak landscape into the even more forlorn terrain of the new Czech Republic. The ice queen of Narnia must have represented *Communism, a brutal system that turned all to stone* and the 'statues' were only slowly returning to life.

Dr. Ivan expressed some concern for me, wrapped his jacket around me and offered to bring me back to the one star-nostar hotel to which we had been assigned and which possessed an abundance of carrots.

The round-about journey was via a taxi driven at high speed by what appeared and sounded like a former KGB hitman, with an array of porn photos on his dashboard.

I had enough of his whirligig navigations and spoke sternly in Russian.

Dr. Ivan looked like he wanted to dive under the seat, but 'KGB' taxi-driver sat up straight and said 'Da,' and brought us quickly and directly to the hotel. The Iron curtain may have fallen, but the 'imprint' of the 'Iron Maidens' of the Soviet underbelly was still as chilling as the landscape.

At the hotel, Dr. Ivan went into over drive. He insisted on bringing warm drinks to my room, brought extra blankets, and decided he should stay to 'observe' in case I developed a fever. He sat in an armchair as I fell asleep for.

'Ivan' fell asleep too, in his armchair until…

We awoke to a banging on the door.

Had KGB come to exact revenge?

"Don't open it!' said Dr. Ivan.

"Dr. Ivan! Dr. Deirdre! Are you in there!"

It was an American voice. One of our company. I was about to open the door, but 'Dr.Ivan' grabbed my arm.

"Don't open it!" he pleaded, "someone might tell my wife!"

"Tell your wife what?" I asked, puzzled at his newly manifest panic.

"That I, that I…"

"That you fell asleep helping a friend - besides who, here, knows your wife?"

Most of the company, it seemed.

"But what if someone is sick and needs you or I? Besides, they will come to their own conclusions anyway with *both* of us unavailable…"

"I will say we went to a nightclub…"

"That's better?"

"You don't understand," he said.

"You're right," I thought, "I don't."

The following morning at the breakfast of carrots, er, rolls and coffee, carrots and more carrots, as I entered the carrot room from one direction, and he from another, seating himself at a different table, there were a few interested glances, brief and polite.

One of the group leaders came in, saw us, and came over to me. Mrs. 'Beauregard' was ill last night. We were looking for you.

'Mrs. B?'

A stout, reticent mature woman with dark brown hair, unhappy since her arrival in Germany. She –wisely– took to her room in Prague and was not visible during our walkabout the once glorious city.

"She had some, er, abdominal pain," he said, a good Catholic male highly uncomfortable with 'womens' issues,' - "if she doesn't recover we'll have to bring her to the Canadian Clinic, and stay in Prague for up to three more days…"

"The Canadian Clinic?" I asked to mask my rising panic at the prospect of three more days in the Carrot House Hotel. Did I mention the plumbing? Or the confabulated contraption masquerading as a shower?

"It's the only, er, Western style medical service in Prague. I don't know what you can do, but…"

"No you don't know what I can do," I thought.

"…but will you at least see her?"

"Of course – did you ask Dr. Ivan?"

"Yes."

"Of course, you asked him first…!"

"And?"

"He said he was a paediatrician."

"Interesting," I thought, as the organiser led me to Mrs. B's room and left me there.

She was still in agony – Colon pulse full and bursting, Small intestine pulse tense and wiry; excess yin, insufficient yang…

Mrs. B had been 'blocked' since arriving in Prague, and a few days prior. The bus journey was agony, every jolt painful; In bed, every movement was an effort, and aggravated her pain.

She was quietly assertive, a woman accustomed to her own way, but without being obnoxious. Later I learned that she was an heiress to a 'small' shipping fortune. There was none of the tentative reticence of the *Nat mur* 'tremblors' which would point to the hypernatremic (high sodium) diet of the Bavarian hostel – a four star hotel by contrast with the Carrot House – so I understood that something deeper was going on with Mrs. B.

After asking a few discreet questions, administering the appropriate remedy, and working on her meridians via acupressure, I tip toed out, allowing her to sleep.

The following day she was fully recovered and ready to travel at the scheduled time.

She thanked me and told me to bill her insurance company in New York.

Getting back to Germany was thanks enough.

The bus ride was 6 hours – long enough for me to notice a different kind of 'chill.'

The 'chill' of exclusion by the married women who assumed that the slender New York Homeopathist had seduced the poor innocent Dr. Ivan and 'had her way with him.'

They would make sure 'the trollop' didn't spend the night with *their* husbands!

With good reason! Some of the husbands – who had jumped to the same conclusions – were noticeably warmer after the week-end in Prague!!!

Perhaps in appreciation for their wives' renewed 'romantic interest!' Perhaps not!

I was educated in England where the Royal Motto is:

'Honi soit qui mal y pense!'

Shame on him who evil thinks…or as the Scriptures admonish: 'To the pure all things are pure!

Persons of Faith will appreciate the following anecdote: There was a hold up at the Czech-German border. The bus driver said it could take 8 hours to get through. There were 'industrial' public bathrooms at the border area, so the opened the doors - otherwise we would be stuck on the bus for eight hours – and at European petrol prices, the engine would not be idling.

Another chilly evening and six hour drive in the darkness for a total of 15 hours travel time.

The baby on the bus was crying and crying. Her parents could not get her formula opened, and the small gift kiosk at the border did not have the right opener. None of us had what was, essentially, a 'beer key.' No, they were not feeding beer to their baby! The packaging was unusual, perhaps Czech, perhaps German, probably not American.

The baby's cries melted everyone's hearts. I turned to my immediate neighbours on the bus and suggested that we pray the Rosary.

By the time we had reached the 5th decade (about 10 minutes) the bus driver announced that the blockade had cleared and the bus would be moving within 20 minutes.

He also made a stop on the German side where the parents of the hungry child acquired an opener.

Win win.

For the fearful flier – the rosary is also effective with turbulence. Pretty much anything benign, in fact!

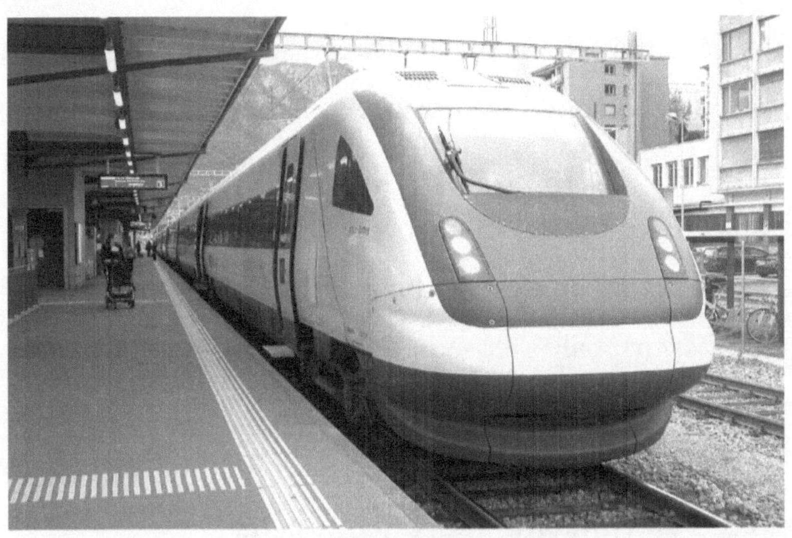

MUNICH – WHEN THE ZUG ZUG MADE A ZIG ZAG!

I was invited to visit a hospital for alternative medicine in Munich. Dr. Ivan expressed a strong interest in accompanying me, so to the alarm of the group, we disappeared for the afternoon. More scandal!

Many German towns have a Bahnhopf and a Stat by the same name, so if you don't know the system you can end up on the wrong express heading toward another region entirely.

We did make it safely to Munich, and while the Medical Director welcomed me cordially, I was disappointed to see that they were not doing the level of work that I had the privilege of attaining in New York.

The work was more maintenance than curative.

Most of the patients whom we saw were suffering from joint disease and had worsened on orthodox medicine. They were mostly out-patients.

I was hoping to see the dramatic and challenging cases that I had read about from the early days of Homeopathy, before Big Pharma spuriously closed down our hospitals and faculties, but was disappointed. It appeared that Homeopathy remedies were used as a *replacement* for orthodox prescriptions, but within the allopathic system.

Still it was good to see a hospital designated exclusively for Alternative Medicine, albeit limited, albeit lacking Hahnemannian Homeopathic protocols.

At Munich the station was large and spotless. On acquiring tickets for our return, the attendant handed us a print out with the name of the train, the carriage numbers, the name, rank and serial number of the gentleman who had painted the train…er no! I exaggerate, but the shadow of the war and the efficiency of the rail network seemed inextricable.

What was totally unexpected was the good nature and *sense of humor* of the German train conductors and station masters, all of whom spoke excellent English, even those assigned to rural stations.

Our conductor had a shaved head and ear-ring and looked rather menacing, but laughed his head off at the final stop when he learned we had missed our destination, now thirty miles behind us.

The amused conductor said he was on a break, but guided us to another train standing by, opened the door, said "Stay here, sit down, don't leave and in twenty minutes I will return and get you back to your station."

We had taken the express rather than the local. One served the 'Stat' station and the other served the 'Bahnhopf,' but you'll have to call Munich to find out which is which. Many smaller stations in Germany are unattended.

I certainly can't tell you, but they will speak excellent English, and they will know exactly what track, number, carriage, etc., that you will need and which station is which.

They just won't know that you don't know that the ticket you are purchasing may be for the wrong train entirely!

The German for train is zug zug. Ours took a zig zag.

Cute.

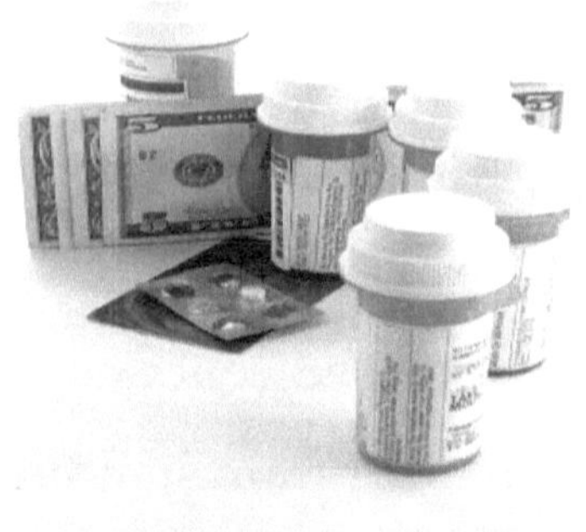

THE PARANOID PEDIATRICIAN AND THE POCKETFUL OF PROZAC

My faith in Homeopathy is such that when I do not get the positive results expected from a carefully chosen prescription, I start to suspect 'interference' from orthodox sources.

'Ivan's' relapses were baffling.

He would be fine after the remedy to the end of day, then disappear into his room until the following morning, when the same worried, harried person would appear again!

At the end of the seminar, the expected transformation from worried, paranoid, suicidal persona to energized, optimistic, life affirming professional had not taken place.

He had assured me that he was not taking any meds, but like every other addict protecting his sources, he lied.

I learned that after our long sessions, he would sabotage the effects by engaging in long, transatlantic diatribes with his distant wife. Usually about money. Or so he claimed.

That was certainly his prerogative, but I started to wonder why he would claim that his marriage was over when it was still very much alive - rancorous, but dynamic, and abuse my therapeutic skills and time, if the relationship had not ended.

I wondered what else he was not truthful about.

He said he could not consult a psychiatrist or see a counsellor about his suicidal ideations because in his State, that would put him at risk of being struck off the register.

But his psych colleagues provided him with ample supplies of unsupervised psychotropes.

He claimed to have discarded all his medications, but his addled confusion, and periodic short term memory lapses suggested otherwise.

Still he insisted.

On the last day of the seminar, I went, for the first time, to his room, to return a book.

It was morning, before breakfast and I tapped on the door. Fortunately another member of the group was observing from her balcony and saw me arriving. Otherwise anyone seeing me emerging from Dr. Ivan's room at that hour would assume the worst.

The taste for scandal in supposedly Christian communities is, in itself, scandalous!

The Dr. opened it, looking dishevelled, even addled.

He seemed frightened, checked the street, like a character in a B spy movie, and ushered me in.

"What if someone saw you coming in here!"

"Someone did!"

"Who? Who?"

I mentioned the lady on the balcony opposite and asked what was the problem.

Before he could answer, my gaze landed on the coffee table which was literally *covered with prescription psychotropes, including a pile of boxes of Prozac – with prescription labels, yet!*

"You should have told me," I said, "I would not have wasted my time and energies…"

"No," he insisted, "You helped me, you really helped me. I am going back to try and make my marriage work. My family depend on me."

I don't like failure. Even when it's not mine. He was still addicted. And Prozac was still complicit in the suicides of its users. Homeopathists need to know *everything – especially if orthodox meds are used to sabotage my work.*

Then again, he had 'sobered' up long enough to rethink his marital status, and no longer saw suicide as the only way out.

The assembled company, each of whom was dealing with different issues, would not return to their desolate Eastern European enclaves, their industrial North American enclaves and their declining European Union satellites with the shadow of the doctor's suicide hanging over them.

Instead, they returned with what they believed to be a juicy scandal!

Oh well!

Whatever floats your boat, as they say in Ireland…

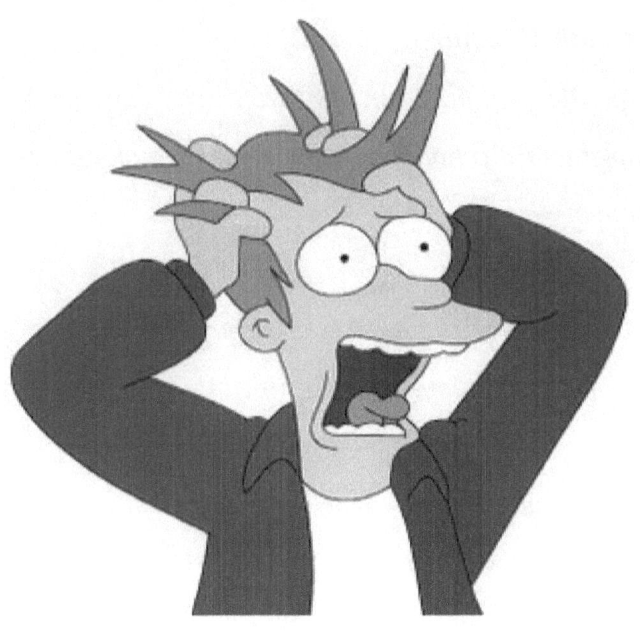

OBSERVATION: Prescription meds and violent crimes.

- *Under the influence of Prozac and a 'moderate' amount of alcohol, a male acquaintance committed a reprehensible felony;*

- *Under the influence of a different psychotrope, another male acquaintance likewise committed a felony.*

- *A female "Church lady" Buspar and Beer abuser abducted a child.*

- *These persons were all reputable persons of good standing in the Catholic Church.*

- *A gentle Buddhist on Synthroid was exposed to marijuana smoke and alcohol and went berserk, violently attacking her spouse.*

From what I know of them, it seems that their medications and/or meds plus alcohol, played a significant role in their aberrant behaviour.

The abuse of psychotropes developed as 'chemical restraints' for persons incarcerated for mental illness must be re-evaluated in a civil world, but until we put the essential God given Human Rights of our people above Pharmaceutical and political profiteering, we cannot claim to be either civil or civilised.

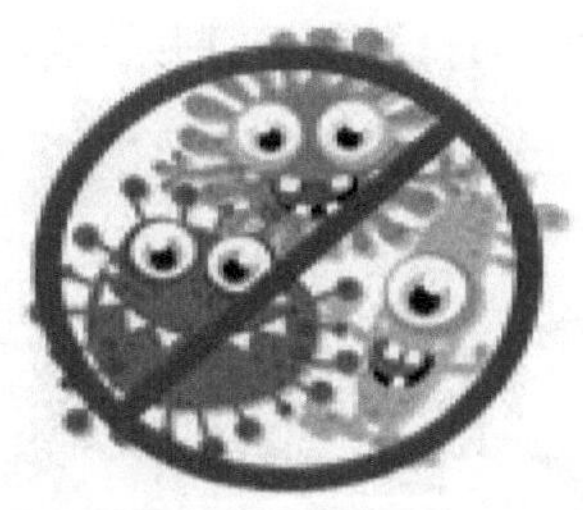

ABC – The Hepatitis Family and Homeopathy.

Hep C – All my patients free and clear of viral load on both sides of the Atlantic according to their labs. Just as pleasing – disappearance of the grey pallor, depression and more personal symptoms accompanying this sad disease.

One of my Hep C patients returned to the allopaths, didn't tell me, but I knew immediately that something was wrong. He was extremely weak and could barely support his own head. Reluctantly he admitted letting his MD give him a Hep B shot, because he was doing so well!

I took the "totality of symptoms" and prescribed accordingly and effectively.

I got a call from Europe from a distinguished artiste. He was unable to work for three months following a bout of Hep A. Could not accept job offers or fly.

Treated accordingly, closely monitored for a week, he was off on his travels within three weeks. Hooray for Homeopathy!

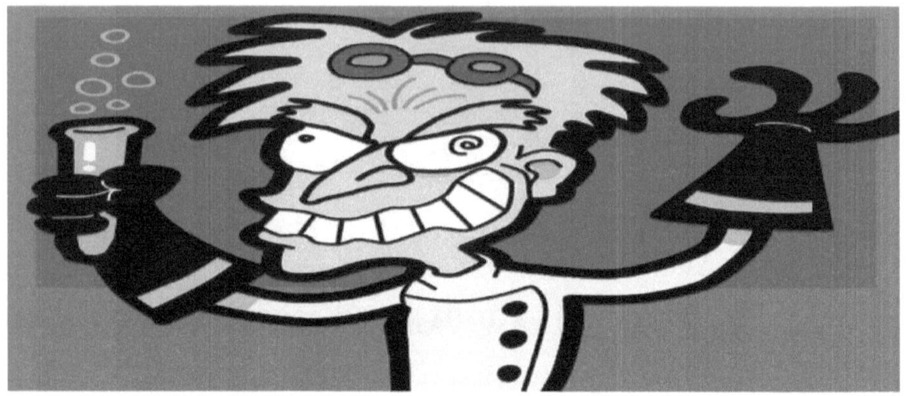

THE ACCURSED VACCINES

How many people must die, and how many children injured and lives ruined before they will put a stop to this diabolical practice?

Edward Jenner came out with the first vaccine a few years after Hahnemann's great Organon, but where Hahnemann's discoveries CURED, Jenner's killed – even his own son, not mention a few of his neighbours.

He was about to give up when Big Pharma stepped in and the rest is history.

Homeopaths have a phenomenal recovery rate in the 1918 flu epidemic – which followed the first mass vax movement and almost 50% of allopaths' patients. (6% of ours and we took the sickest.)

I had the privilege of a call from a dad in England, a lower income dad, desperate to help his child, suffering from multiple seizures since a vaccine. I prescribed according to the totality of symptoms.

The following week I received an effusive and incredulous thank you note from the dear man.

One seizure after the remedy, *then complete cessation of seizures.*

Mass vaccinations create a sickly, Rx dependent population. Homeopaths warned against them from day one. Two hundred years later, we are sadly, proven correct as various forms of "autism" have appeared in the young, along with paralyses (sic) seizures, death, and desperation, and in the elderly alzheimers, parkinsons and death – all following vaccinations.

Always just a "coincidence" that flu season follows so closely on "flu vax" season which is always set up for the Holy Days and maximum interaction and cross contamination.

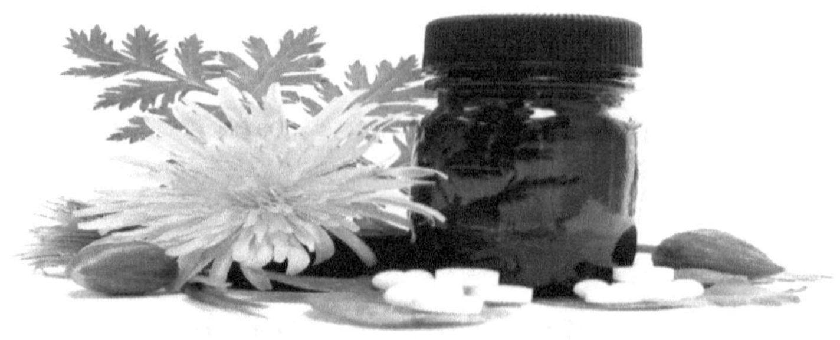

"GREYSCALE" BE GONE!

To illustrate my books, I sometimes use clip art, and sadly, must convert the pretty, colorful photos and drawings into "Greyscale."

It's nice to have that option, but visiting a former patient in Ireland who suffered from glaucoma and had all the orthodox "treatments' I learned that she could no longer see color.

To her, everything was grey scale. To understand this, I asked her to identify the colors in a tapestry on the wall of a business that we visited. It was all gray.

I like a challenge, so prescribed according to the totality of her symptoms and returned to another part of Ireland.

Two or three months later, I returned, and she correctly identified all the colors of the cars of the road, etc., and objects which prior to the treatment would have been a blur.

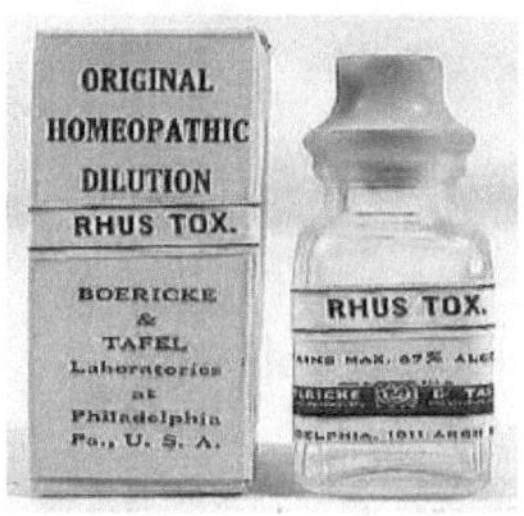

LYME

A gentleman consulted me. He was on disability with Lyme disease and the classic symptoms.

Within six months he was driving a taxi and enjoying life, free from symptoms.

OCTOGENERIAN WITH OSTEOPOROSIS

Gracious lady, 84, with osteoporosis fell and fractured her humerus, or upper arm.

Under Homeopathic care, it healed completely within three weeks. This is on record at Bellevue Hospital.

Female, 60s, sustained double fracture rescuing an active six year old. No cast, just a boot. Horrified the orthopaedist by walking in 3 weeks later without said boot. Homeopathic care again.

So many diseases, considered "incurable" have responded rapidly to Homeopathy, but we are only as effective as our patients "allow" us to be. Work with us and be hopeful.

We need full symptom pictures, a clear field and no interference from intermittent medications, unless that is agreed upon and factored in prior to the commencement of treatment.

Nil desperandum. There is always Hope, Homeopathy and Miracles!

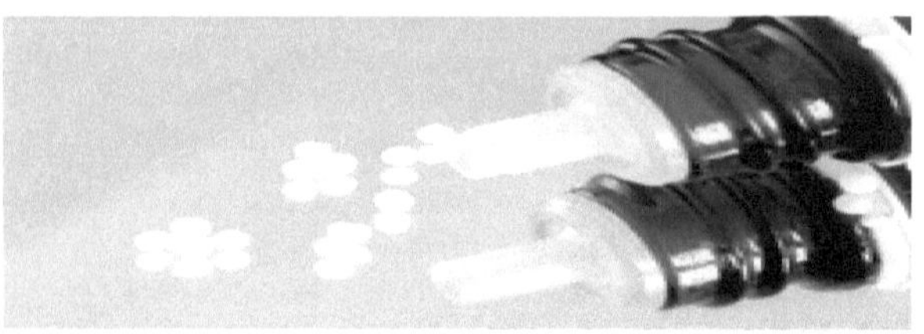

THE PIETISTIC PEDOPHILE

From time to time I would volunteer with a youth group in a low income area of NY. There I encountered a young man, seemingly steeped in prayer and piety, whom I had seen at other youth assemblies.

He asked if he could come to me for counselling, said he didn't have the means to pay.

Although he had wealthy benefactors who offered him scholarships and paid for his transportation to various events in Europe, I agreed to treat him *pro bono.* He had some physical problems where I hoped to put Homeopathy to good use.

He survived a sad and tragic childhood. Signed his soul away to the occult in his teens. Said he had reclaimed it and converted his life.

That was the first session.

When he arrived for the second session, he was challenging, combative. I could work with that and through that.

I could not work with his triumphalist declaration that he attended the youth events and conferences to gain access to young Hispanic boys as he marched out the door for the last time.

The youth group was so advised. For the safety of the children, first, then for his own safety. If the older brothers of the targeted children learned of his intent, the pietistic pedophile would be floating down the East River minus a body part or three.

Mandated reporting is the law. Sometimes the law is, as Mr. Micawber (Dickens character) says, an 'ass.'

Sometimes it can inhibit a search for guidance or clarification. Sometimes it makes sense and saves lives.

Here, I hope it had the intended result, but with his slew of well to do patrons and clerical psychologist friends to defend him and vilify the 'New Age' Homeopath, he may still be on the loose.

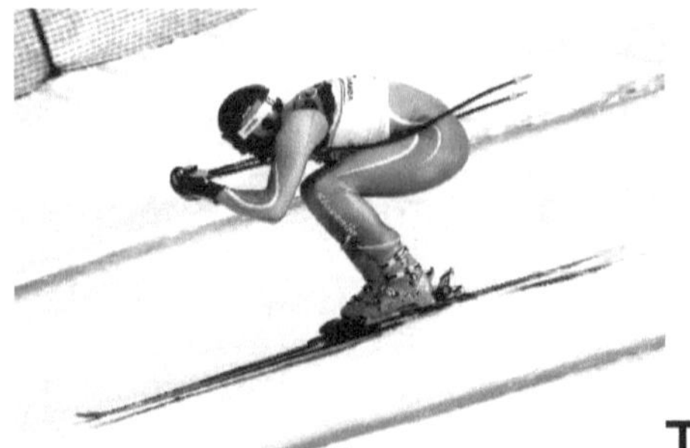

THE PEEVED

PULMONOLOGIST

We 'does our best,' so to speak, and when a distinguished Ivy League friend and Cardio Pulmonary Surgeon continued to limp months after a sprain on the ski slopes I offered to help.

With a giant dose of scepticism he accepted my assistance – as a challenge and with a bet against his own recovery.

Needless to say, I won the bet, but instead of being happy he was peeved to the hilt!

An honourable man, however, he coughed up and while we've lost touch, I believe we are still friends!

And, as far as I know, he is still skiing!

As Oscar Wilde once put it – 'There are no grateful people, only resentful ones!' Partly true, indeed, but sad for Oscar. I know mostly appreciative, loving patients, whom I see as Gift and for whom I am eternally grateful.

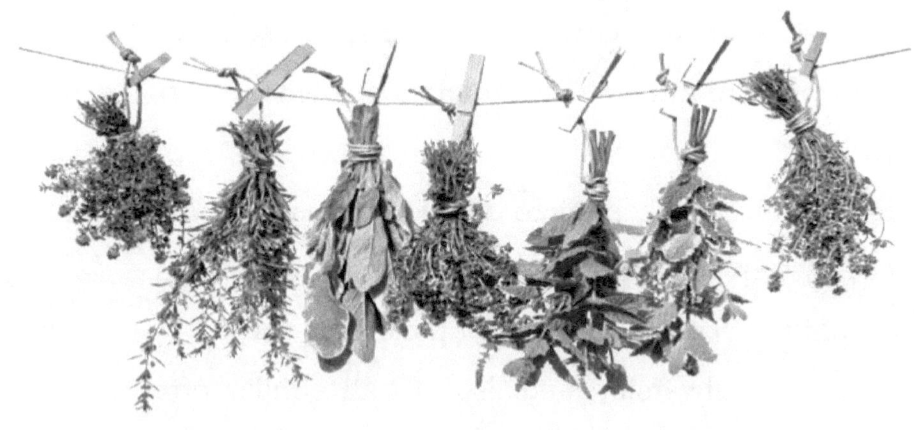

THE BAFFLED BIOLOGIST

Going 'off piste' where rules are concerned, I made some recommendations for the close friend of dear friend and advocate of Homeopathy, a woman whom I admire greatly.

Her male friend was a biologist who suffered from severe sinusitis and a variety of plant allergies.

His condition improved considerably.

Of course, being a biologist he wanted to know the "whys" and "wherefores."

As many well-meaning people believe that Homeopathy is something found in 'Grandmother's kitchen,' there's a cognitive dissonance of cosmic proportions between popular impressions and our experts' opinion that it 'takes 10 years to make a Homeopathist.'

He was baffled because the remedy used was indeed 'something found in Grandmother's kitchen.' In it's raw, untriturated form.

However, it had been micro diluted, succussed or 'dynamised' at every step and stage, 'proven,' then 'proven' again.

It could then create an 'echo' of the effects caused by over use of the material version, and also cure all 'similar' effects.

Years ago, when Homeopathic remedies were all but impossible to obtain in NYC, the usher at St. Patrick's Cathedral walked me and my young son to the front row, just as Cardinal O'Connor ascended the pulpit to preach the Easter Sunday Homily - and just as my young son started to sneeze and sneeze and sneeze, in complete harmony with the late, great, Cardinal O'Connor, who did not, however, bat an eye.

No withering glances from *his* pulpit! I knew him as one of the kindest, most patient and tolerant men on the planet.

The front row was decorated with a huge bank of *Azaleas*, but we were blocked and could not leave.

He also suffered from hay fever and cat allergies, and Homeopathic remedies were extremely difficult to locate in NY.

When I returned home, I took samples of all the plants in my courtyard, pollen if possible, leaf where not, and along with an azalea petal from the Cathedral prepared a 3x dilution, and administered a few drops.

For the next three summers, no allergies. By that time, Commercial Homeopathic preparations became available in New York.

As an adult he can walk in the woods with impunity and has three cats, no allergies!

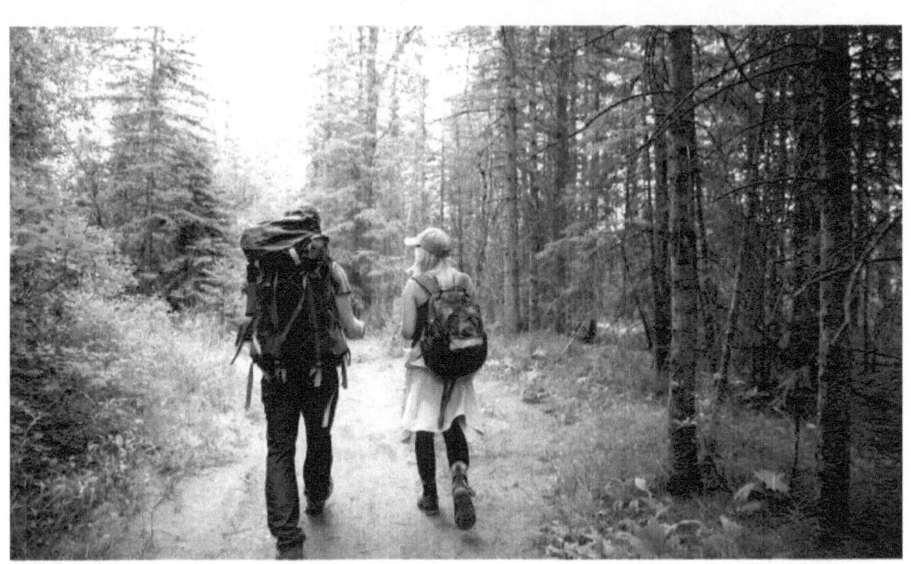

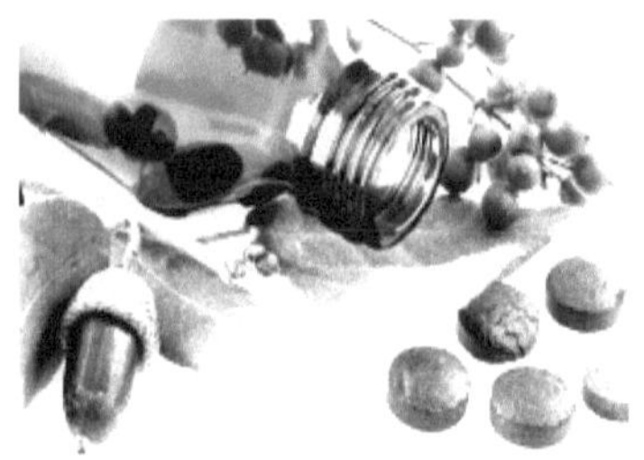

THE ENEMY WITHIN?

The late, great, Cardinal O'Connor opened the door to Homeopathy at a Catholic Hospital.

He arranged a meeting between the female Director of Health and Hospital Services, whom I found cold and hostile and her cohort; myself, Dr. John Vecchione, Medical Director of Goldwater Memorial Hospital, and Thierry, the scion of a European Homeopathic Pharmaceutical Company.

The Cardinal was not present at this meeting.

As cold as the Director was, I was not prepared for the blatant sabotage by the heir apparent of said Pharmaceutical Co.

He was the first in his family line to study Business rather than Pharmacy, so even if his heart wasn't in Homeopathy, he should have recognised the incredible opportunity when it presented itself to him.

I often wonder what agreement was made between Big Pharma and the FDA to confound and confuse the general public in regard to our praxes.

Making the remedies widely available was a blessing, but the benefits were somewhat "antidote" by the instructions for use on the blue tubes and in the pamphlets, instructions derived from allopathy, and not consistent with basic principles and praxes of Homeopathy.

Some of our blessed remedies can be used by the general public, if they are properly advised that "less is more," and not given carte blanche to use remedies that require deep study, comparison and complex analyses to use correctly. This is why I now hear: "I tried Homeopathy but it didn't work."

It doesn't take long to ascertain that Homeopathic remedies were used, but used incorrectly by agreement with the FDA!. "Goal" – FDA! "Own goal" – America!

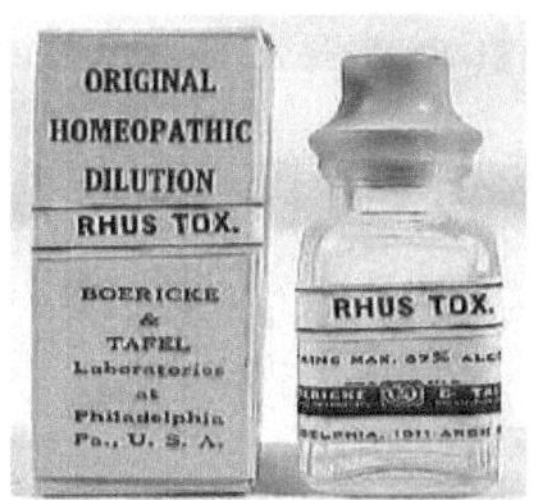

HOMEOPATHY and THE GAMALIEL PRINCIPLE

There's a dark side to being a Homeopathist in practice. That is, some consider us to be 'outside the law,' unstructured, anything goes, New Age, so to speak, when, in fact, Homeopathy is Western - German in origin; refined, challenging, rigorous, intrinsically law abiding. In England, we have a Royal Charter – by reason of the Homeopathic cure of Haemophilia in Queen Victoria's grandchild.

We are sought out by heads of State, Medical Specialists, and even Pharmaceutical executives – who then turn around and promote the dangerous and uncalled for mass vaccinations of vulnerable and low income populations.

Good for the oul' municipal pension funds! You cannot serve God and Mammon!

We are also get the occasional call from friends of friends of friends with mysterious injuries; from Mid Easterners expecting us to make house calls in the middle of the night, and from parents, desperate to reverse vax injuries. Yes, we can do a lot for many of those poor children, but few know to call us.

All the Royals, to my knowledge, enjoy robust health now, courtesy of Britain's fine Homeopathists. The contrast between the presence of haemophilia on the German Hanovers' family tree and that of their British cousins is one of the best affirmations possible of Homeopathy's profound genetic impact.

To those who take the time to really study it, and understand Hahnemann's inspiration, its impact is so awesome that one wonders if a 'Divine hand' is protecting it from profane users.

After all, one does not have to dig too deep to see how degraded medical and bio science has become. The authentic and ethical practicum of Homeopathy gives us a profound insight into the human condition in general and our patients in particular.

The average life span on the Homeopathic practitioner is 85 years, according to Dr. Marjorie Blackie, late Homeopathist to HRH Queen Elizabeth, noting that many of said practitioners come to Homeopathy via the failure of orthodoxy to effect positive change in their own chronic ill health.

The average life span of the orthodox allopath, is 65 years. That may be extended in recent decades, since they have adopted so much of our lateral health enhancement recommendations.

Taking the bathwater, but ignoring the 'baby!'

The Cinchona bark which provided the 'Eureka' moment for Samuel Hahnemann, apothecary and doctor, came from Peru. It was named for the Countess of Cinchon, a benefactor of Surgeon and Saint Martin de Porres beloved poor. St. Martin gave it to Jesuit missionaries who gave brought it to Rome, thence Germany, where became known as *quinine.*

Baffled by a friend's prolonged quotidian (daily) fevers, and prolonged ill health, Hahnemann noted that the symptoms expressed by his friend corresponded to symptoms caused by the over use of quinine. His, friend, however, had not used quinine. Hippocrates, Galen, Pliny, often speculated on what Hahnemann later termed the Law of Similars, ie, 'that which causes, cures,' or 'Like cures Like' and administered quinine to his friend, with spectacular results.

He then closed his practice and gathered the finest physicians in Leipzig to embark on the most intense investigation of the properties of plant, animal and mineral life *ever* to take place on this planet.

This was not publicly funded. Nor was it a private, profit embarking enterprise. It was pure dedication to the service of human kind.

Needless to say, human kind has not yet paid Hahnemann his dues, even refusing to acknowledge the *explosion* that took place within orthodoxy in response to Hahnemann's published findings.

Jenner, Pasteur, Semmelweiss, Freud, and other notables, took inspiration from his work, but picked and poked, and sometimes, distorted his discoveries.

Fortunately for the world, top Ivy League graduates got together, formed the first professional medical body in the United States, and formed The Society of Homeopaths.

This was followed a few years later, by the American Medical Association, or AMA, funded by Big Pharma with the sole intent of suppression Homeopathy.

If it is from God, it will prevail. Gamaliel principle.

It's from God.

It prevails.

That we practice 'on the fringes' sometimes, is more reflective of the greed and lawlessness of a Pharmaceutical Industry that prioritises profit over patient, and spends a fortune to demean other, time proven healing systems – *at the expense of humanity, even while recalling one product after another.*

So much for the highly vaunted 'double blind test,' which cannot be applied to Homeopathy, any more than it can to acupuncture.

In some ways, however, our seemingly marginalised status can put us in a position of discovery, as shadowy figures appear in our waiting rooms, or at the other end of a phone line.

They believe that we are outside the law, like themselves.

Sometimes that makes someone more comfortable in expressing sorry or anguish; other times it becomes a "license" to bully and /or attempt to manipulate.

For instance a male with a pronounced Mid-East accent somehow acquired my unlisted home telephone number and called me, around 7 pm, insisting I drive out to Yonkers – about thirty miles away – and treat, for no fee whatsoever, a 'friend.' A friend who could not go to the Emergency Room or see a doctor. He would meet me at Yonkers Station and drive me the 'rest of the way.'

Not only was he a complete stranger, miles from NYC, but he was aggressive and angry, with a bizarre sense of entitlement. When I told him that I would have to pay for a bodyguard, he went berserk. "Nobody else, nobody else!'

Right! 'Not enough money in this world, not enough money in this world,' to walk into what seemed to be the world of subversive jihad.

A few months later a call from a female with a Mid East accent – what could I do for snake bites in the desert…

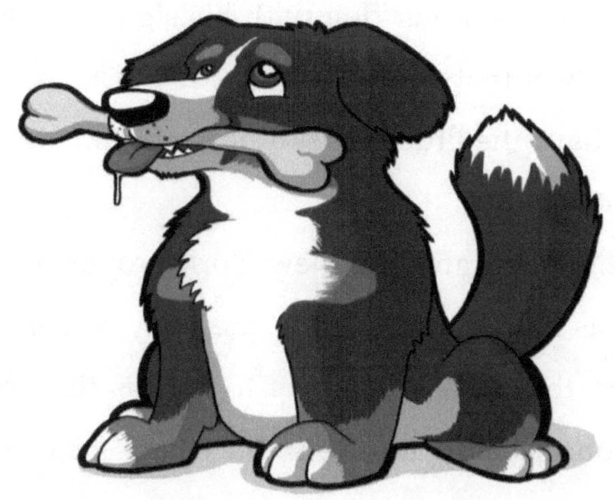

MARY HAD A LITTLE DOG – OR THE BEGINNING AT THE END

My first patient after I re-opened my practice in New York was an amazing woman.

While she was a registered patient, I would like to pay tribute to her, without violating her confidence. This is not about her condition or health status.

She had the voice of an opera singer, a powerful mezzo soprano, and the heart of an angel.

She loved babies, children, life and 'creatures great and small' and dedicated her life to the care and protection of the vulner able.

She asked if I could help her dog with his sight, but that was beyond my ability at that point.

She refused to have the little dog put down but knew he only had a few months to live.

Winter was imminent, and the New York ground would be frozen. She was not about to throw the body of her lifelong companion into the trash, preferring to see his final place of rest where he once chased squirrels and where she could visit after his passing.

The care she took of the little fellow was heart-rending and exemplary; so many children, spouses, patients, could use that level of care and attention. Indeed, the world would be a far far better place if my friend Mary's heart was 'the norm.'

It isn't.

We devised a strategy whereby Mary and her friend would go into the park at night, with a flashlight, dig a little by his favourite tree, stuff plastic bags in the cavity, and cover it with a sheet of ply-wood, grass and twigs – easier to remove than frozen mud.

After a couple of nights, the tiny grave was ready. They were not disturbed by any patrols or busy bodies.

Mary returned to her tender care of the little dog, and one icy December morning, called to say that her faithful companion had died, and that she and friend had buried him under his favourite tree, and that all had gone as planned.

She took the loss well, being a person of Faith, and soon her apartment was filled with other happy animals, rescued from shelters and lonely, unloved death by injection.

Her example is humbling.

Ad multos annos, Mary!

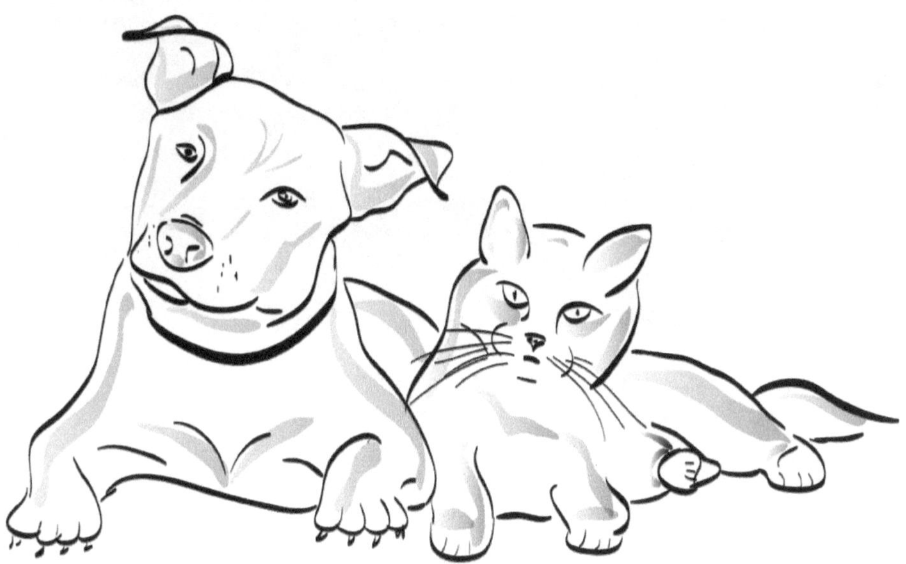

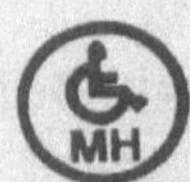

GOLDWATER MEMORIAL HOSPITAL
NEW YORK CITY HEALTH AND HOSPITALS CORPORATION
FRANKLIN D. ROOSEVELT ISLAND, NEW YORK 10044
TELEPHONE: (212) 750-6800

12/28/93

To whom it may concern:

________ a patient at Goldwater Memorial Hospital has a diagnosis of Cerebral Thrombosis with left hemiplegia, dysarthria and dysphagia. He has also CAD for which he has had by-pass surgery. He has had multiple problems with urinary tract infections and aspiration pneumonias. His multiple antibiotic regimens have given him funguria + fungemia.

I took the liberty to ask Dr. Deirdre Mc Namara to see him in consultation. She is a homeopathic practitioner and has been seeing him since October 1993 on a weekly basis.

The patient is now stronger, off his ventilator and afebrile. His urine has remained clear without antibiotics, he has gained weight and is being considered for diaphragmatic stimulation for his central sleep apnea.

Medical Director, Respiratory Care

John Vecchione, M.D.

We love the challenging cases, the relief of suffering, especially bringing hope to the "hopeless." Such a privilege to be the first Homeopath in a century to consult in an NY Hospital. Thank you, Dr. Paul Vecchione, Medical Director of Goldwater Memorial Hospital!

AN FYI TO INSURANCE PROVIDERS AND ELECTED REPRESENTATIVES:

Within a few months of treatment, one patient was transferred from a labor intensive Respiratory Unit, where he had lain for 18 months, into a Nursing Home Unit.

The savings to Insurance Company and Taxpayer was $1,000,000 per year.

It is also my professional opinion that had they not used him experimentally after his wonderful initial recovery, the cost to the Insurance Company and Taxpayer would have been $0.00 within a year, if not six months.

Crash courses for your MDs will *not* be effective in complex cases. Acupuncture is now a neutered protocol. We will not permit Homeopathy to be minimised like that.

Homeopathy must be treated as a respected and challenging specialty, *under our own auspices and aegis.*

For the *serious* student:

Remedies used in the vignettes:

Arnica Montana
Arsenicum Album
Bryonia
Causticum
Cocculus
Histaminum
Natrum Muriaticum
Nux Vomica
Rhus Toxicondren
Ruta Graveolens

Of General Interest:

Homeopathy was developed in the late eighteenth century by Dr. Samuel Hahnemann of Leipzig.
He was a qualified physician and pharmacist.
The great Greek physicians, Hippocrates, Pliny, Galen, all pondered the principle of 'Like curing Like,' ie, symptoms caused by herbs that were also used to cure similar symptoms when unprovoked by said herb.
When his friend fell ill with quotidian fever, Hahnemannobserved that his symptoms were similar to those of quinine poisoning.
Quinine used to be called Cinchona. Cinchona bark was discovered by Surgeon-Friar St. Martin de Porres who named it after the Countess of Cinchon, a benefactor of his beloved poor.
He sent it to Europe via Jesuit Missionaries where two centuries later it became the foundation for the most thoroughly researched, most profound and most effective form of healing the world has ever seen, the dynamic therapies of HOMEOPATHY!
The publication of his pivotal work, 'The Organon' was met with awe, fear, fascination, respect, and horror by arrogant profiteers preying on the sick. It inspired an explosive response – giving orthodox medicine new fields of study – immunology, nutrition, genetics, psychosomatics, and new, kinder treatments for the sick and suffering. Like it or not, Jenner, Breuer-Freud, Semmelweiss, Lister, et al all followed Hahnemann – but could not completely cross over. Jenner killed his own son and many neighbours with vaccines; Lister gave us antisepsis which lead to the "sterilization" of the body with antibiotics as well as the environment. We like asepsis.

Semmelweiss insisted on cleanliness and was initially persecuted by the surgeons of his time, whose prestige was proportionate to the amount of blood they wiped on their already encrusted jackets as they spread puerperal fever from one mother to another.

Many did, follow Hahnemann faithfully, however, and in the USA, The Society of Homeopaths was the first professional medical body, attracting top students from the Ivy Leagues. Homeopathy was used effectively in the Civil War, and in the 1918 global 'flu' epidemic – a 'flu' developing from the poverty, horror, deprivation, malnutrition, stress, lack of shelter, destruction, fear that followed WWI and the Bolshevik Revolution. Homeopathy's patients had a remarkably higher survival rate than orthodoxy despite allegedly getting patients dumped out of orthodox's hospitals. In recognition of which, Homeopathy's patients received discounts from New York's Insurance Companies! Longer lives, better health, fewer complications!

Contact: Deirdre McNamara 8001 Castor Avenue, 521, Philadelphia, PA 19152. Service: 215 588 5251
celticbalm@yahoo.com

THE TUSCANY EXPRESS" IS DEDICATED TO THE GREAT HAHNEMANNIANS PAST AND PRESENT - GRATITUDE TO DR. MARGARET TYLER, DR. MARJORIE BLACKIE, GREAT ENGLISH WOMEN HOMOEOPATHISTS - AND TO MY DEDICATED FRIENDS IN ORTHODOXY, WHO SHARE THE SAME DESIRE TO RELIEVE HUMAN SUFFERING. ABOVE ALL, TO YOUNG NICCOLO.

SIMILIA SIMILIBUS CURENTER![2] Let likes cure like!

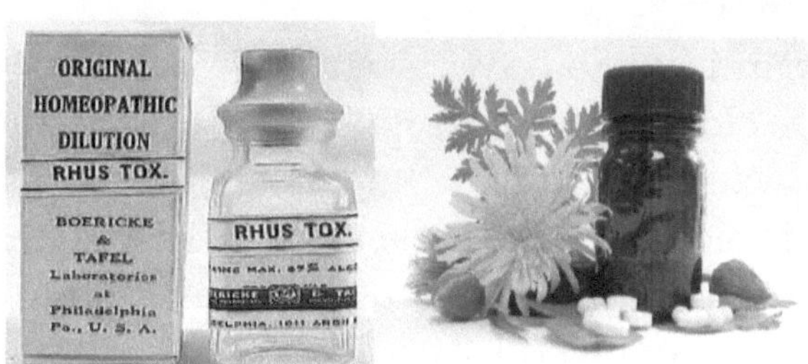

About the Author:
Let likes cure like!

Deirdre McNamara discovered Homeopathy after a childhood and adolescence of protracted illness and misdiagnoses.
Homeopathy cared and Homeopathy cured!
She embarked on an extensive study and opened a practice in New York City where she became the first Homeopathist in almost a century to consult professionally in a New York Hospital.
She particularly honors Dr. John Vecchione, former Medical Director of Goldwater Memorial Hospital for making his patients' well-being a priority and for inviting her to embark on a research project using Homeopathic protocols to wean patients off respirators.
The proposal passed six committees, and was headed for final review at NYU when New York's near lethal anti Life politics 'intervened.'
'The Tuscany Express' – Scenes from the Life of a Homeopath will hopefully show how effective and gentle this intensive therapy can be.
Before primitive assay, spurious science and political corruption closed our hospitals – Homeopathy had the best statistics. We still have the most thoroughly researched Materia Medica and the most dedicated practitioners though we are largely excluded from the professional, financial and social supports enjoyed by orthodoxy.
However - according to the late physician to HM Queen Elizabeth, Dr. Marjorie Blackie, MD, Homeopathist, we have the greatest longevity!
And a Royal Charter in England.
To your good health!

LIST OF BOOKS AUTHORED BY DEIRDRE MCNAMARA, HOMEOPATHIST AND DRAMATIST

Most are available from Amazon.com and Kindle.com

NEW CHRISTMAS STORIES FOR CHILDREN

THE SANITY OF CHRIST vs THE FALLACIES OF FREUD

SOS – For Survivors of Suicides

CHILD SEXUAL ABUSE – Never Call It Love

MEDITATIONS ON THE MYSTERIES OF THE ROSARY – A dramatist's view of Christ's life

THE DEMISE OF SENATOR DUFF – Fiction. Corrupt Irish politician meets a bitter end. Whodunnit? Plenty of suspects - you decide!

THE TUSCANY EXPRESS – Use of Homeopathy in travel emergencies. 'Lite' - under revision

CELEBRITY CITY – Unexpected encounters with NY's celebrities.

THE FAMINE REPORT – Irish Famine eye witness reports in dramatized form.

THE DISGUISE – Set at Christmas and based on The Prodigal Son.

NIC and CATULA – Abandoned kitten and sad little boy 'rescue' one another. 4th grade and above.

TOM and the HAPPY CAT – for very small, sick children.

TOMAS AGUS AN CAT SASTA – as Gaeilge (same)

IN PROGRESS: Three more

IN RESCUE:

HIC EST QUIES MIEA;

SUMMER OF THE DISCONTENT;

HOMEOPATHY – GIFT OF A GRACIOUS GOD;

THE MAN IN THE MOON MADRIGOL; *

FUGUE ON AN AMERICAN THEME (Four parts) etc*

MANY DRAMAS, PRODUCED AND IN WAITING.

ONE OF THE HUNDREDS OF
METICULOUSLY RESEARCHED

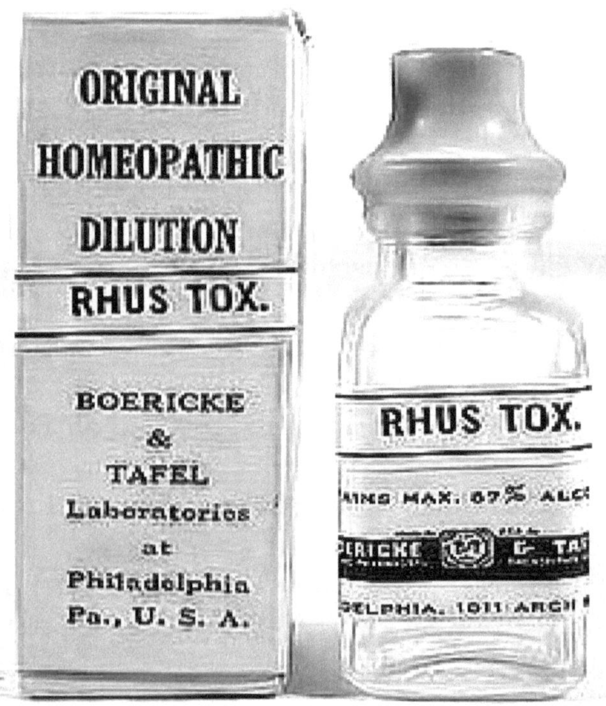

GIFTS OF A GRACIOUS GOD!